Intermittent Fasting

*The Ultimate Beginners Guide for Weight
Loss, Burn Fat, Heal Your Body, Cure
Illness With Intermittent Fasting and
Ketogenic Diet*

KATHLEEN MOORE

i

Table of Contents

the owners themselves, not affiliated with this document.

Introduction

Congratulations on downloading *Intermittent Fasting : The Ultimate Beginners Guide for Weight Loss, Burn Fat, Heal Your Body, Cure Illness With Intermittent Fasting and Ketogenic Diet* and thank you for doing so. Making the decision to take control of your weight loss once and for all is a difficult one and should be applauded. Unfortunately, it is only the first on a long road, one that intermittent fasting can make far easier.

Fasting is a tradition that is older than even the written word. While using it as a method of weight loss is a relatively new phenomenon, it has long been used for numerous other purposes including to commune with the divine, prevent disease, reduce the signs of aging, enhance concentration and more. Fasting has been used by virtually every religion and every culture since the time that agriculture made the question of when the next meal was coming in obsolete.

With all of this in mind, the following chapters will discuss everything you need to know about intermittent fasting and how you can get started as quickly and effectively as possible. First, you will learn all about the ins and outs of intermittent fasting, what it means and the benefits you can expect from doing it regularly. Next, you will learn about many of the misconceptions surrounding intermittent fasting as well as how to separate fact from fiction. From there, you will find half a dozen different types of intermittent fasting, virtually guaranteeing that you will find one that is right for you. You will then learn about intermittent fasting and exercise as well as additional tips and tricks for success.

The second part of the book then concerns itself with helping you take your weight loss to the max by introducing intermittent fasting's natural partner, the keto diet to the mix. You will learn about why these two great habits go great together, as well as how to add the keto diet to your new intermittent fasting habit without missing a beat. You will then find a variety of recipes chosen to illustrate the types of delicious foods you can expect to enjoy once you make the switch to the keto diet. Finally, you will find additional tips for sustaining the choice in the long-term.

While every effort has been made to ensure the information in this book is correct and as relevant to as many people as possible, it is recommended that you speak with a nutritionist or healthcare professional about your personal dietary needs before making any major dietary change. There are plenty of books on this subject on the market, thanks again for choosing this one! Every effort was made to ensure it is full of as much useful information as possible, please enjoy!

Chapter 1: Intermittent Fasting Basics

Intermittent fasting is a way of eating to ensure that you get the most out of every meal you eat. The core tenants of intermittent fasting mean that you don't need to change what you are eating, instead, you have to change when you are eating it. Intermittent fasting is a viable alternative to traditional diets and can help fasters lean up without changing the number of calories they consume in a day. In fact, the preferred method of intermittent fasting is to simply eat two large meals every day instead of three (or more) meals in that same period of time.

Intermittent fasting is also a great option for those who traditionally have trouble sticking to diet plans as it only requires you to change one small habit instead of several larger ones. Intermittent fasting is extremely effective for most people because it is simple enough for them to attempt yet effective enough to actually warrant doing. The key to understating why intermittent fasting is so successful lies in the differences in your body during a fasted state versus a fed state and the important changes that will come across as a result of changing your dietary habits and sticking with it.

The body is considered to be in the fed state when it is in the process of absorbing and digesting food. The fed state tends to start roughly five minutes after you begin eating and then lasts for anywhere from three to five hours depending on how long it takes your body to digest the meal. A fed state, in turn, leads to higher levels of insulin in your system which make it much more difficult for the body to burn fat. The period directly after the fed sate is referred to as the post-absorptive state which is the period of time where the body is not actively processing food and its insulin levels begin to fall. This state lasts for between eight and 12 hours and directly precedes the fasted state.

The fasted state begins somewhere between nine and 12 hours after the post-absorptive state, which is the point where your insulin levels will have bottomed out. This is also the time when the body will burn the most fat during physical activity if you train it to do so by following the keto diet as suggested in the later chapters of this book. Unfortunately for most people, they rarely wait so long between meals which means that regardless of whatever else they may be doing to lose weight, they aren't burning fat as effectively as they might otherwise be. Luckily, if you are eating too frequently with your current lifestyle, you can build more muscle and burn fat more quickly by simply altering your eating habits a little bit.

Clinical studies

Many studies have been done on the effects of calorie restriction (low-calorie diets) on the health of humans and animals, but the effects of intermittent fasting on humans, where caloric restriction has occurred on a strict schedule, has not been widely clinically studied.

One study that was performed by Martin, Mattson, and Maudsley (of the United States National Institutes of Health) in 2006 indicated that the effects of intermittent fasting on health are similar to those of low-calorie diets.

Both calorie restriction and intermittent fasting put stress on cells, which brings about resistance to metabolic and environmental stress without doing any harm.
Calorie restriction and intermittent fasting also increase insulin sensitivity and reduce glucose and insulin levels.

Intermittent fasting studies performed on animals by Mark Matteson, senior investigator for the National Institute on Aging, showed that the animals who were subjected to intermittent fasting experienced better learning abilities, memory, reduced oxidative stress and showed improvement when it comes to combating diseases.

Studies performed on humans showed that the body goes to fat stores for energy somewhere after 10 to 16 hours of fasting. Not surprisingly, the studies also showed that the body starts to quickly bring down a person's weight when a person combines intermittent fasting with a low-calorie diet that consists of quality food.

Mr. Mattson thought that perhaps the body resists disease because fasting puts the body's cells under mild stress, which brings about adaptation the stress. This is what the body does when a person exercises.

Additional benefits of intermittent fasting

Reduces inflammation in the body: Oxidative stress is hard on the body and it can be one of the risk factors that come with aging and other chronic diseases. This kind of stress is going to involve a lot of free radicals, or molecules that are considered unstable, reacting with some of the important molecules that your body needs. These important molecules can be things like DNA and protein in the body. When the free radicals react with the important molecules, they will end up causing damage.

There have been several studies that show how intermittent fasting is a great way to enhance how your body resists oxidative stress. In addition, there are other studies that talk about how intermittent fasting is important for fighting off inflammation. Inflammation can be hard on the body because it is going to be the key force behind many other harmful diseases in the body. With the help of intermittent fasting, you can effectively reduce the amount of inflammation that is in the body and get your health back on track.

Fights diabetes: Furthermore, traditional intermittent fasting, as well as alternate-day fasting, are medically approved ways of minimizing the risk of developing type 2 diabetes in those who are already suffering from pre-diabetes. Both of these types of fasting are known to help glucose levels return to normal in as little as 12 months. This benefit can be negated, of course, if the practitioners of intermittent fasting use the fact that they are fasting as an excuse to eat anything and everything during the periods they are not dieting strictly. This is folly, however, as the best way to see long term results is to not treat fasting as something special and to instead think of it as just another part of your daily routine.

To study fasting's astounding efficacy on the human body, an experiment was performed using yeast cells which found that generating an artificial food scarcity for the yeast caused its cells to start dividing slower in response. This literally means that while fasting, each and every one of your cells lives noticeably longer than would be possible with the lack of scarcity.

Remember the most common consequence using this procedure is hunger—not starvation. You might experience some mood swings and want to over-eat when you are on your days off, but the plans are healthy.

Starting off strong

With so many compelling reasons to give it a try, it is understandable if you are chomping at the bit to get started. In order to make sure you can stick with the type of intermittent fasting you ultimately choose, however, there are a few basics you should keep in mind first.

Eat less than you burn: While the concept of burning more calories per day than you consume is hardly a new one, it is nevertheless important to bring it up here as it is far easier to overeat on an intermittent fasting plan than it is with most other diets, especially early on. Slipping during one post-fast meal could well be enough to undo all of your hard work for the day.

Don't forget, there are 3,500 calories in a pound of fat which means you need to burn at least this many per week in order to keep up what is considered a healthy amount of weight loss in the long-term. While you will likely see more than this for a time, it is considered a health risk if this degree is kept up for too long.

Ensure you remain in control: Another vital part of intermittent fasting is ensuring you can remain in control of your hunger, even when it is at its peak. This means it is extremely important that you have the right relationship with food right from the start. If you are the sort of individual who feels as though specific foods have an unavoidable pull over you, then you may find it especially difficult to get started on the intermittent fasting plan once and for all. Don't forget, it is vital that you go a minimum of 12 hours without eating if you want to start seeing benefits, and any influx of insulin resets the clock. Furthermore, you need to cut out 500 calories per day if you want to lose a pound of fat per week.

While doing your best to avoid eating at the wrong times is key to intermittent fasting success, it is only half of the battle. For some people, having the willpower to start eating again within the healthy-eating window is just as difficult. If you intend to make intermittent fasting part of your life in the long-term then it is vital that you learn how to add it to your life in a healthy fashion as going too far in one direction or the other is only going to lead to failure and potentially serious health problems.

Build a lifestyle: When it comes to getting the most out of intermittent fasting possible, it is important to try a variety of options at first and then plan on settling in to a long-term routine that works for you. Unlike many diets, the true benefits of intermittent fasting aren't felt in the short-term at all, and starting and stopping all the time is only going to slow things down even further. While you will start off seeing some benefits, it will likely take about a month for your body to fully adjust to the changes you have made which is why it is important to commit up-front as nothing happens overnight.

While the going is sure to be tough at first, once your body learns when it can start to expect calories regularly you will find that your overall level of hunger basically returns to normal. After about a month you should begin to see the physical benefits of fasting as well, which should make it even easier to commit in the long-term.

On the contrary, if you make the mistake of only using intermittent fasting for various short bursts, then as opposed to enhancing your natural ability to lose weight and build muscle, it will instead be far more difficult for you to be successful as your body will be in a constant state of confusion. If you hope to see quality results in both the short and long-term then you need to find the right schedule of eating that works for you and stick with it no matter what.

Talk to a professional: While intermittent fasting certainly helps people build muscle and lose weight, in addition to a variety of other health benefits, this doesn't mean it is going to be the right choice for everyone, right now. Potential side effects during the transition period include things like constipation and diarrhea, which will put it out of the reach of some individuals. Likewise, binging can lead to internal damage. Regardless of how healthy you plan to be, it is vital that you talk things over with a healthcare professional or a dietitian to ensure that you don't accidentally end up doing more harm than good.

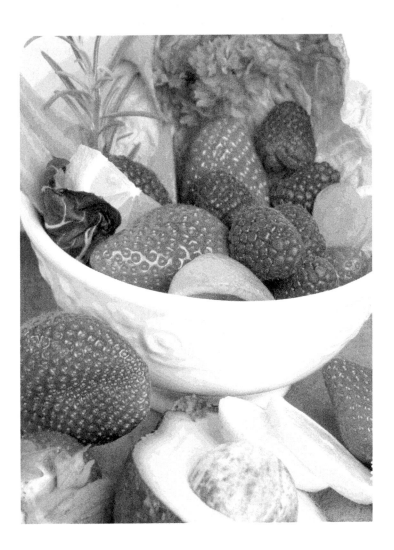

Chapter 2: Clearing Up Intermittent Fasting Misconceptions

While the science is certainly there to back up the claims made by intermittent fasting enthusiasts, the simple fact that the habit deviates from what conventional wisdom dictates has caused many people to make negative assumptions about it without doing their homework first. This, in turn, has led to a wide variety of misconceptions that this chapter is going to endeavor to clear up so that you can get started finding the type of intermittent fasting that works for you with a clear understanding of exactly what you are getting yourself into.

Myth 1 – Only a select group of people can use intermittent fasting without issue: This is one of the most commonly held misconceptions when it comes to intermittent fasting and is one of the leading reasons many people never make the effort to see if it will fit their lifestyle. This is quite simply not the case, however, especially as it is common these days for many individuals to adopt a schedule that is closer to intermittent fasting without their knowing. This tracks with what most people who fast regularly like about the process which is that it can easily fit into almost any lifestyle.

Consider the fact that, for many people, the day starts as late as possible which leads to a rush out the door, a small lunch in the early afternoon, a larger dinner and then probably a snack before bed. If this is a schedule that you follow, all you need to do is check the times you are eating a little more closely and you are already prepping your body to take advantage of all possible intermittent fasting benefits. With breakfast currently out of fashion, you will find getting in the habit of fasting regularly easier than you might expect.

What's more, this pattern of eating serves as a natural counter to the bloated, over-full feeling that most people get when returning from at 12 pm lunch as intermittent fasting is guaranteed to leave you feeling far less lethargic come lunch time. In fact, considering how busy the average schedule is these days, the added benefit that intermittent fasting saves time, as well as money, means that it is easy for virtually anyone to get started on.

Myth 2 – Intermittent fasting is just a cover for an eating disorder: While purposely withholding from eating might seem like an eating disorder to some people, the truth is they are ignoring the mentality of the faster and only focusing on the aspects they see as troubling. In order to successfully continue to fast intermittently in the long-term, the person fasting needs to carefully monitor their eating habits, ensuring they get plenty of nutrients from the foods they do eat in order to ensure they don't get sick. This mindset is completely different from that of the person with an eating disorder who gives no care for the state of their body or their long-term health.

What's more, if you look at the number of calories that a person following an intermittent fasting diet is consuming you will see that they are not restricting their calories any more than any other diet, they are just going about the process in a different way. The simple truth of the matter is that it can be easy to see the worst in any diet that you are unfamiliar with, but they are typically pretty healthy as long as none of their practices are taken to the extreme.

Finally, there is no type of intermittent fasting that recommends anyone goes more than 36 hours without food, which is 12 hours outside of the point where most people will start feeling the negative effects of not eating. Similarly, it is constantly stressed that those who are finishing a fast muster up their self-control and take things slow when first starting to eat to give the body time to adjust to receiving food once more. All of which goes to show that intermittent fasting only looks like an eating disorder to those who are looking to draw that conclusion.

Overall, it is far more beneficial to place the true emphasis on the number of calories that an individual consumes in a given period of time as opposed to the time of day at which those calories were consumed. If you look at the number of calories a person who is fasting consumes in a week, as opposed to someone on any other calorie-restricted diet you will find the same results.

Likewise, to say that just because the person who is intermittently fasting is binging because they are eating a large meal is to miss much of the underlying reasons and symptoms associated with eating disorders. There is nothing inherently unsafe about eating a larger than average dinner to meet your caloric needs in a controlled manner and it is something you will become very accustomed to as you try out the various types of intermittent fasting available.

Myth 3 – Eating your largest meal right before bed is a great way to lose weight: While this can certainly be true for some people, the logic behind the issue is where this myth comes to light. The truth is, it doesn't matter how much you eat, or when, it matters how much available energy your body already has available. As most people are constantly providing their bodies with more carbs than they could ever need, all that happens when they eat before bed is that all of their leftover energy gets converted to fat to be used later, in case of an emergency that is unlikely to materialize.

On the other hand, those who are following some type of intermittent fasting plan don't have to worry about excess energy reserves, which means that anything that they add to their bodies before they go to sleep will be used up long before there is enough left over to turn into fat. As long as a person who is fasting intermittently is making the effort to ensure they are getting enough nutrients, they should have no reason to be afraid their healthy meals are going to mysteriously become fat.

The *Singapore Journal of Medicine* recently confirmed this to be the case by studying Muslim women during Ramadan and finding that they still lost weight despite the fact that nearly all of their daily caloric intake came from one nighttime meal. This study is just one of many that proves there is little difference when calories are consumed as long as your body is in a state to put them to work.

Myth 4 – Intermittent fasting leads to muscle loss: This myth stems from the assumption that if one is not consuming protein every few hours then the body immediately enters a catabolic state where it starts to break down its muscles for energy. This hypothetical issue is compounded by the fact that it does not have the tools it needs to repair/build and maintain muscle tissue. While there is some science to back up this idea, it only holds water if the person in question went into a fasted state without taking the proper precautions (eating a meal before doing so.

In fact, slower digesting proteins, such as casein, take as many as 20 hours to digest fully which means that a person who is fasting for 16 hours per day is still receiving fresh fuel when it is time to eat once more. In fact, it is not uncommon for those who plan on exercising during their fast to consume more than 100 grams of slow-digesting protein prior to starting their next fast.

The thing to keep in mind here is that extended periods of fasting certainly would cause some muscle loss due to de novo gluconeogenesis kicking in after liver glycogen and amino acids are depleted, however for people who are fasting intermittently who generally eat a large, balanced meal before fasting again, neither of these situations is likely to occur in any meaningful degree with the fasting times discussed in the next chapter.

Myth 5 – Intermittent fasting affects performance: While it is certainly true that a person would perform more poorly at the gym if they attempted an intense workout without the proper preparation, there is no reason to assume that your performance would be affected if you take the proper precautions to start with. In fact, studies were done on athletes who train during Ramadan show as much. They show that that both aerobic and anaerobic performance remain unhampered by intermittent fasting as long as the athlete maintains the proper level of nutrients and adjusts their training time to match their meal structure. As intermittent fasting doesn't limit water consumption there is no chance it will negatively affect athletic performance.

This is not to say that when you start exercising while fasting that you won't feel as though something is off, only that this is a mental block as opposed to a physical hindrance. If you feel sluggish, hungry or weak when training while fasting, if you give yourself a week or two to adapt to the change, then you should find that those subjective signals pass and your performance returns to where you expect it to be. This is only if you decide to train while fasting, to begin with, of course, which is hardly a requirement as most types of fasting provide you with plenty of opportunities to adjust your schedule accordingly and train only when you are not fasting.

Myth 6 – The fasted state is the same as starvation: This myth is likely at the heart of a wide variety of the myths discussed here and it stems from the fact that, in today's world, where food scarcity isn't a thing most people ever have to think about, the word starve is often used rather loosely. Simply put, fasting is not starvation unless you are using it as a cover for something much less healthy. Fasting is a conscious choice that you have complete control over which means you determine when it starts and when it ends.

If a person is literally starving then they have been unable or unwilling to find food past the point where their body is starting to be worse for wear because of it. This is not a conscious choice and they have exhausted any means of avoiding the state, not choosing it willingly. Unless you are already living uncomfortably close to this line then you are not going to reach this state if you follow the guidelines discussed in the next chapter.

The difference between the two states can even be seen at the metabolic level. Once a person enters a true starving state, the body shuts down all non-essential processes which are why being in that state is harmful in the first place. As a result, the metabolism drops as low as it possibly can go. In contrast, while the body is in a fasted state, remember the metabolism increases which is what causes the increased weight loss in the first place. Down versus up, polar opposites, fasting is not starving.

This myth is also related to the idea that intermittent fasting can lead to malnourishment which also assumes that you are already malnourished, to begin with. While there was certainly a point in time in human history where it was important to eat as much as possible because it was difficult to determine when another nutritious meal might materialize, those days have long past. As long as you are taking the proper precautions when you are not fasting, and as long as your diet includes plenty of healthy fruits and vegetables, then you have nothing to worry about when it comes to malnourishment in the short or long-term. Regardless of what type of fasting you choose to pursue, as long as it is done safely, you will replenish anything you lost with your next meal.

Myth 7 – Intermittent fasting can lead to low blood sugar: This myth is a bit easier to forgive as those who are first getting started with intermittent fasting can sometimes experience a state that is similar to hypoglycemia as their bodies adjust to their new way of eating. A mixture of cortisol, low glycogen levels, and insulin resistance can cause symptoms similar to low blood sugar but they will go away on their own if the fasted state persists. It can be tempting to eat something sweet in the moment, but it is far better to let the body sort itself out in the end.

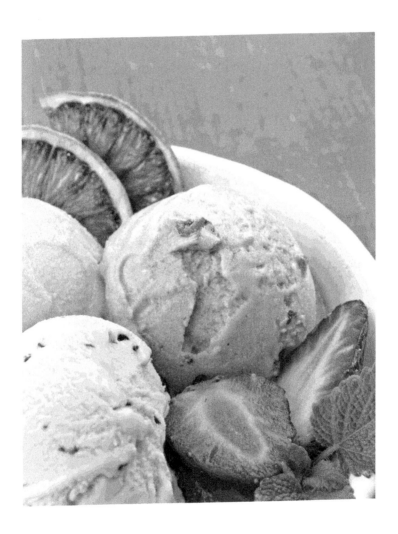

Chapter 3: Types of Intermittent Fasting

While the facts that cause intermittent fasting to be effective are universal, there are multiple variations on the process that helps it work itself into practically any schedule. Many of these vary in intensity, as well as the meals that they include or exclude, which means you are statistically likely to find one that fits your daily schedule while also allowing you to easily attain your fitness and weight loss goals.

In order to find the right type of fasting for you, you will want to try each of the following types of fasting for at least a month to give your body the time to respond properly to the differences found within. You don't want to shift directly from one type of fasting to another either. For the best results take at least a week to eat normally in between different types of fasts to give your body a baseline to return to as you find the type of fasting it responds to most readily.

Eat-Stop-Eat Method

Brad Pilon is credited with developing this method of Intermittent Fasting, and he did so because he was tired of all the problems people had with rebound weight gain. Each time they would diet and somehow manage to drop to their goal weight, in a short while they'd pack it all back on again—and then a few pounds more.

Pilon is an international author and nutritional expert who set out to prove that intermittent fasting didn't work, that fasting gave false promises. However, all the evidence he uncovered pointed to a different hypothesis. He soon discovered his mistaken beliefs and began to experiment and research a new fasting method that would benefit people who felt they had nowhere else to turn. That when Pilon developed the Eat-Stop-Eat method and offered hope to thousands of individuals all over the country.

What Pilon discovered was that people were stuck in a rut because they believed what they had been told by trusted scientists and renowned nutritionists, as well as hungry product advertisers and marketers all those years. They believed what many people still believe, and that is that if you just had enough self-discipline, you can take the weight off and keep it off. There's a problem with discipline, though. When most people begin dieting, they have enough discipline in reserve to get a good start, but it soon wanes and leaves them with nothing but ravenous hunger in its place.

If you're like the people Pilon studied, chances are you have similar beliefs. The frustrating cycle of taking the weight off just to put more back on is not your fault any more than it has been for the millions of others who tried before you. Only two percent of those who lose weight manage to continue to keep it off after all.

With Pilon's intermittent fasting method, you eat normally five days a week and then fast for either 20 or 24 hours the other two days. For example, you would eat dinner on Tuesday and then eat breakfast again on Thursday. You will want to schedule your fasting days at least two days apart from one another to give your body time to recover from the strain of not eating for 24 hours. The caloric intake on the days you are not fasting should be about 2,500 for men and 2,000 for women.

On the days that you are fasting, you will want to limit yourself to water, diet soda, tea, and coffee. On the days you are eating regularly you are going to want to feel free to eat what you will, within reason. Make it a point of adding plenty of high quality fruits and vegetables to your diet. Additionally, you are going to want to aim for at least 200 grams of protein per day to give yourself enough to ensure that your body continues functioning properly during fast days. Aim for 50 grams every three to four hours. Using high-quality protein powders to ensure you hit this amount is recommended. If you feel as though you are still gaining weight, consider cutting out more carbs on non-fasting days.

Some people will not be able to adapt to such a strict type of fasting, you will know that it is not for you if you continue being irritable during fast days after a month or so and if you continue to experience periods of dizziness or headaches. With that being said, the benefits to this intermittent fasting method are undeniable and it offers the freedom to alter when you are fasting based on need. Whatever you do, however, it is important to never fast for two consecutive days and never fast for more than two days in a single week.

With this fasting method, it is essential not to fall into a habit of fasting and binging because it will create havoc within your body. This type of intermittent fasting is only for those with the self-control to prevent themselves from falling into an unhealthy eating cycle as a result.

You should engage in an exercise program along with the Eat, Stop, Eat plan. Instead of cardio, such as walking, running, jogging, or swimming, the plan prescribes high-intensity resistance and weight-lifting to build muscle. This should be done three to four times a week, almost every day that is not fasting. You don't need to exercise on fasting days. Recommendations are that on non-fasting days, you do six to 10 reps of two to four different exercises per body part. The exercise routine is designed to supplement the fasting regimen to help you lose as much fat and gain as much muscle as possible.

Try a minimal yoga session or light cardio exercise if you are completely 'out of it' on your fasting days. Any more vigorous exercising could make it difficult to achieve the time allotment of your fasting schedule. Remember, at first it is common to feel angered, anxious, fatigued, or have headaches. This will pass once your body adjusts to the new dieting plan.

Fasting 16/8

As the name implies, in a 16/8 fast (also known as Leangains) men go 16 hours without eating and women go 14 hours between meals and then eat normally for the remainder of the day which is anywhere from eight to 10 hours. This period can then either comprise three smaller meals or two slightly larger than average meals that should be filling, while still being health conscious. During the majority of the fast, all you should allow yourself are carbonated beverages that contain 0 calories, unaltered water, gum which contains no calories and coffee, but only if you are comfortable drinking it black.

Of all of the types of intermittent fasting discussed in this chapter, 16/8 fasting is one of the most flexible as it can be adapted to fit any schedule. Additionally, two larger meals in an eight to 10-hour span is enough to leave the average person feeling completely full for about 12 hours which means you then really only have to get your body used to not eating for those remaining four hours.

Most people who follow this practice typically eat two meals during their eight or 10 hour period as well as a snack or two. The important thing here is to find a schedule that works for you and stick with it so that your body can learn when to expect food and when to stay quiet.

This type of intermittent fasting typically begins after dinner and then lasts until lunchtime the next day when the cycle starts all over again. This doesn't mean this is the only way this type of intermittent fasting works, however, and in fact, one of the best parts of intermittent fasting of all types is the ease with which a schedule can be altered should the need arise. As an example, if you typically exercise soon after you wake up in the morning, then you may want to break your fast earlier in the day so you can fuel up after you work out to ensure your body has what it needs to build new muscles. It is recommended that you don't spend any part of your eating time asleep.

Regardless of the timeframe you choose, it is important that it works with your body's natural inclination as opposed to being something that you have to actively struggle against. Your goal here should be to follow the same eating habits every day as this will also serve to maximize your overall results as well. If you mix up your fasting timeframe with too much regularity you could end up disrupting your hormones and making it far more difficult to lose weight than it would otherwise be.

This type of intermittent fasting is ideal for those who plan on exercising while fasting as it means you will still be consuming enough food every day to not really have to worry about holding back on your existing exercise routine as long as you take it easy during the transition period. If you plan on truly giving it your all then you are going to want to work to always break your fast with lots of dark green leafy vegetables, nuts, and seeds. When these are consumed in tandem they combine to give you a serious shot of energy along with the protein you will need to make it through the day. Keeping your energy levels up throughout a fast can be tough but if you make it a focus then you should be able to find something that works for you without too much trouble.

Generally speaking, your best choice is going to be breaking your fast with an average meal before exercising within the next four hours and then eating another larger meal as soon as you are finished with your workout. During this larger meal, you will want to focus on consuming enough complex carbohydrates to power yourself through the next day. By making a concentrated effort to fuel up fully, you will be able to make Leangains a part of your life in the long-term.

If you do not plan on exercising quite so much when on the Leangains plan then you will want to add in additional healthy fats instead of protein. If you are aiming to lose more than 20 pounds then you will need to watch what you are eating carefully in order to ensure that you are bringing in at least .7 grams of healthy fat per pound of body weight in order to see the best results. Regardless, you should go out of your way to avoid simple carbs, unhealthy fats, and processed foods and focus on natural alternatives whenever possible.

Assuming you then plan on mixing in some exercise as well, then you will want to be aware of the numbers you are striving for every day to ensure that you don't accidentally overeat on the days you aren't exercising. In order to ensure you maintain steady weight loss then you will want to consume about 60 percent of your total calories during the first meal and the rest during the second meal. This should be switched on the days you plan on exercising.

5:2 Fasting

The 5:2 diet is another effective option that you can choose to go with. With the 5:2 diet, you will be allowed to eat normally for five days of the week. Then on the other two, you must restrict yourself to eating between 500 to 600 calories for the whole day. These two fasting days should not be consecutive, or it is not that effective, but otherwise, you are able to pick the days that work best for you.

When you are on your fasting days, the calorie restrictions will be different for men compared to women. It is recommended that women eat no more than 500 calories and that men eat no more than 600 calories. A good example of this diet is that you would eat normally each day of the week except on Mondays and Thursdays. On those two days, which are your fasting days, you would consume a pair of meals that are 250 to 300 calories each. You do not have to go with Monday and Thursday for fasting though; pick out the two days that are the busiest for you and make those your fasting days.

The 5:2 diet plan is pretty accommodating and flexible, with limited restrictions. You can pick when you want to eat and when you would like to fast depending on a schedule. It is more flexible compared to other methods when it comes to altering fasting and eating times.

Here comes the big catch now, especially for those who have not fasted before. Going off food for an entire day can be challenging if you are just getting started with intermittent fasting. This is more challenging for people who are required to perform demanding tasks through the day or those with families to look after (preparing meals for children).

Another flipside is that you have to caution against the trap of overeating after fasting for a long duration. Feeling ravenous after fasting for 24 hours may make you overeat, which may not really support your weight loss goals in addition to being damaging to your body.

Alternate day fasting

Yet another intermittent fasting protocol is the alternate day fast. This specific protocol requires that you eat regularly one day and then fast the next day. You are allowed to eat any food that you like on your non-fasting days. This particular protocol can be modified so that you only have 500 calories on your fasting days.

The alternate day diet is often touted as the most effective form of intermittent fasting in regards to weight loss. Overweight and obese adults who follow this approach have been shown to lose as much as eight percent of their body fat in two months. Middle-aged people, a population that tends to particularly struggle with weight loss, seem to particularly benefit from this program. Much of the fat loss is the dangerous belly fat that can lead to heart disease and inflammation. The weight loss benefits of the alternate day diet may actually supersede those of traditional calorie-cutting alone.

People who follow the alternate day diet and exercise regularly have been able to lose up to twice as much weight as those who merely cut calories. That figure goes up to as much as six times more weight loss for individuals who follow the alternate day diet and exercise, as opposed to those who only exercise. Again, exercising on fasting days may be difficult, especially at first. You may find that the best plan for you is to exercise twice as much on regular days and either not exercise or exercise a minimal amount on fasting days.

This is the ideal fasting protocol for anyone who desires to lose weight. It is very effective because of the frequent calorie restriction throughout the week. Your eating will only be restricted for half the time. For the rest of the time, you will enjoy your meals normally. On your fast days, you are allowed to have all sorts of beverages including green tea, coffee, or water. All these should be calorie-free.

You can modify this protocol so that you consume only 20 to 25 percent of your daily caloric requirements. This is equivalent to 500 calories per day. Studies show that women prefer this form of calorie restriction because it lasts for only a day and they get to choose the foods they want to eat the following day. Traditional diets often require deprivation almost every day and restrictions regarding food choice.

The benefits that you stand to get from this protocol are very similar to the benefits of all the others. Therefore, one protocol is not superior to others and the approach is rather similar. The differences are only a matter of preference and choice.

The following meal will supply you with roughly 475 calories—depending on the type of soup used.

- ½ cup cooked chicken cooked without the skin and topped/Lemon juice/Fresh-ground pepper

- A bowl of tomato or low-sodium vegetable soup

- 1 ¼ cups of fruit salad

For men only: You can have a whole-wheat roll (medium 96-calorie) for a total of 566 calories.

Prepare the salad with pears strawberries, mandarin orange segments, and melon.

Enjoy lean beef: Choose a lean piece of beef cut similar to sirloin or tenderloin steak, and enjoy some low-cal side dishes. The basics of the plan are charted for a woman; for a man—add 80 additional calories with a one-cup serving of asparagus with a teaspoon of olive oil for the topping.

For the remainder of the meal, enjoy a three-ounce seared steak with some onions. Top it off with a bit of blue cheese. Serve it with one cup of chard sautéed in 1 teaspoon of olive oil along with a ½ cup of polenta (cornmeal). Use some lemon juice for seasoning.

Substitute with seafood: You need to consume some omega-3 fatty acids to remain heart-healthy. For men, boost the counts to 553 by enjoying one cup of kale that has been sautéed with olive oil for an additional 102 calories. Flavor the kale with crushed red pepper, red wine vinegar, and garlic.

As a woman (451 calories) enjoy three ounces of sautéed shrimp with jalapenos, garlic, onions, and some tomatoes (fresh and diced) on a bed of ½ cup of brown rice. Place it all in a six-inch corn tortilla. Also, have ¼ of an avocado (chopped) for dessert.

The choice of no meat: Women can choose a meatless meal with 473 calories using a whole-wheat pizza crust. As toppings use some black beans, diced tomatoes, barbecue sauce, fresh corn, and shredded mozzarella cheese. Have a bowl of butternut squash soup made using ¾ cup of fruit sorbet and veggie stock.

Men can veg-out with one cup of cauliflower salad for an extra 48 calories using reduced-fat mayonnaise. He could also add ½ cup fruit such as blueberries, ½ cup yogurt if desired. It is best to use the lower fat plain yogurt with the meal.

Warrior Diet

The Warrior Diet suggests that people are at their very best when they eat less or fast during the day and eat more at night. During the duration of the day, you will mainly be fasting. The fasting period is roughly 20 hours each day. While it is called the fasting period, it is technically more of what is called an "under eating" period. During the fasting period, it is acceptable to eat very small portions of fresh fruits, vegetables, and proteins, as well as drinking freshly pressed juice from the whole foods (fruits and vegetables). Also, during the fasting cycles, your body is releasing human growth hormone, and the body is much more likely to use fat for fuel.

This plan was formulated by fitness expert, Ori Hofmekler, who studied how the lean and muscular ancient Romans and Spartans ate. The ancient

Romans and Spartans ate very little during the day and then feasted on the food they hunted during the evenings. If body building is your thing, this should be your intermittent fasting diet of choice.

More Growth Hormone: As with the full-day fast, a fasting period of 20 hours lets you get many benefits from improved and increased levels of growth hormone in the body. And just as with all types of fasting, you will end up consuming fewer calories over all.

More flexibility with what you eat: This style of fasting offers a unique benefit, which is that you only have one big meal and what you have for that meal doesn't need to be as strict as it would when you eat more often. Getting enough protein and nutrients is important, but your body will handle less healthy foods with much more ease this way.

The beauty of simplicity: It's hard to argue with the ease and simplicity of the warrior diet. When you just eat once per day, it leaves you a lot of freedom to schedule your day however you want, focusing on work, hobbies or time with friends. You also have fewer opportunities to screw up when you know you can only eat one time. For those new to intermittent fasting, starting out simple can be the key to getting comfortable with this pattern of eating and finding what works best for them on an individual level.

What to eat: Remember, this is not an actual water-only fast, but rather a way to significantly restrict your intake during the day and maximize your energy building foods for your nightly meals. For the first 10 to 18 hours during the day, you should limit your foods to light servings of vegetables and fresh fruits. If you feel it necessary, you may include some yogurt as well. It's not about starving yourself, just eating wisely and reasonably. If you are feeling particularly strong, you can do a water-only fast during the day. However, leave this method to a time when you are a more seasoned faster. If you have medical conditions, always consult a doctor.

When you break your fast at night, you must eat particular food groups in a particular order. First, you eat broth, then vegetables, protein/meat, and then fat. You can eat carbohydrates at the end of your four-hour feasting period if you are still hungry.

Eating at night maximizes the parasympathetic nervous system, which helps the body to recuperate, become calm, relax, digest while the body uses the nutrients for growth and for repair. It may also help the body to produce fat-burning hormones that work on your fat the next day.

Foods to avoid: The Warrior Diet advocates the belief that certain combinations of foods slow our digestive track, reduce our energy level, and create a buildup of toxins in our bodies that prohibit us from active weight management. Here are some foods that should NEVER be combined.

- Raisins, nuts, and chocolate such as those things you find in trail mixes.
- Wine and pasta dishes
- Peanut butter and jelly
- Bread and butter
- Honey, nuts, and granola.
- Potato and sour cream.

Forever fat loss

The forever fat loss type of intermittent fasting combines aspects of several different intermittent fasting methods to form something rather unique.

What's more, you even get a cheat day each and every week. To balance out this cheat day, however, immediately following it you are not allowed to consume anything save water, diet soda, black coffee, tea, and 0 calorie gum for 36 hours. You are also allowed to eat a single serving of dark, leafy green vegetables after 18 hours. The remaining days of the week are then split between the 16:8 method and the warrior method.

Fasting for 36 hours straight is automatically going to make this type of intermittent fasting off limits for some people as it is pushing the boundaries of what the human body can handle without starting to take damage from lack of food. Furthermore, the variety of the days means that you are going to need to have a semi-flexible schedule to account for the various differences. Additionally, you are going to need to limit your physical exercise to a minimum on your long fast day in order to get through it successfully.

When you make it to the end of your long fast, you are going to want to start with just a small meal to ensure you aren't overeating and also to get your digestive processes moving naturally after the absence of food. If you find that you have a difficulty controlling yourself during the fast, or that you feel the need to eat a large meal when you break your fast as opposed to a small one then this is likely not the most efficient form of fasting for you. Your goal when fasting, regardless of the type of intermittent fasting that you choose, is to find a healthy and long-term dietary plan which means that if any part of the process causes you to act in an unhealthy fashion then you need to check yourself or focus on a different intermittent fasting method instead.

However, if you can make it through, Fat Loss Forever boasts that it helps users lose the last stubborn five to 10 pounds. It also leads to rapid weight loss; while conventional wisdom suggests that people trying to lose weight should aim for one to two pounds per week, Fat Loss Forever boasts that it can help people lose 10 or more pounds per week. The creators claim that the weight loss is pure fat and, as opposed to losing water weight, which comes back as quickly as it is lost, this fat will be gone forever. It promises these results based on the premise that this intermittent fasting plan will actually reset your body's fat-burning hormones so that you will burn through fat without even trying to or realizing it.

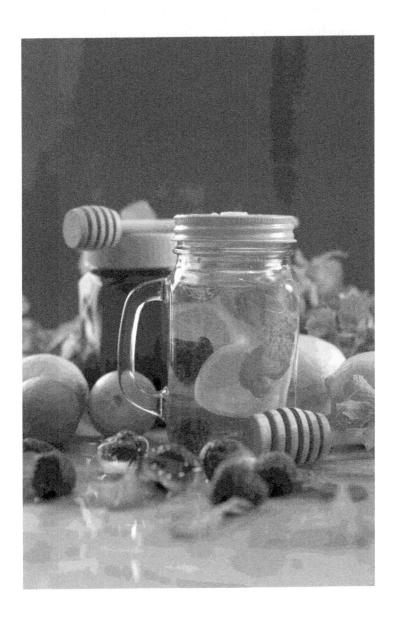

Chapter 4: Intermittent Fasting Concerns for Women

By now you probably understand what intermittent fasting is all about and its benefits for weight loss and your overall health. As a woman, there are a few additional things that you need to know because fasting can affect you in ways that are different from men.

Many women who have tried intermittent fasting acknowledge its numerous benefits. These include reduced risks of heart disease, gaining lean muscle, recommended blood sugar levels, reduced risk of chronic diseases such as cancer and many others.

Potential concerns

Hormonal changes: However, women need to be aware of hormonal changes within their bodies and how these changes are affected by fasting and an active lifestyle. The major concern often has to with women's fertility hormones and fasting. Fortunately, this concern has been adequately addressed, and women can safely fast.

In women, calorie restriction due to lifestyle changes like fasting can alert the body to interrupt fertility. If you ever find yourself going a prolonged period of time without eating (more than 36 hours) you will find that your body adopts a defensive mechanism which is only discarded when sufficient nutrition intake resumes. While fasting can affect your hormones, intermittent fasting does support proper hormonal balance leading to a healthy body and weight loss the right way as long as you don't overdo it.

The hormones responsible for important bodily functions, such as ovulation, are highly sensitive to the energy you consume. In both women and men, the HPG (hypothalamic-pituitary-gonadal) axis, the collective process of three crucial endocrine glands, controls important functions.

Let's look at those now. The hypothalamus in the body releases a hormone that tells your pituitary gland to release another hormone. This hormone acts on the ovaries or testes. For women, this process triggers progesterone and estrogen which is necessary for supporting pregnancy and releasing mature eggs (also known as ovulation). For men, this stimulates sperm and testosterone production. Since this reaction occurs with women in a very specific cycle, these pulses need to be timed, or it can throw it out of sync. These pulses are highly sensitive to factors in your environment, meaning that fasting can throw them off.

Even fasting for say, three days in a row, can throw off some women's hormonal pulses. There is some reason to believe that missing one meal during the day can put women on alert, helping their bodies stay responsive to energy changes just in case this continues. Perhaps this is the reason why some females will handle intermittent fasting fine while others might have issues.

Nutrition deficiency: When adopting an intermittent fasting lifestyle, the first thing women need to keep in mind is that the transition phase is likely going to interrupt the body's natural fertility cycle. This is a defensive mechanism that is only discarded when an adequate level of nutrition intake resumes. While fasting can affect your hormones, intermittent fasting does support proper hormonal balance leading to a healthy body and weight loss the right way once the body adjusts to the new way of eating.

Additional challenges: While it is not something that is going to affect everyone, some women who regularly practice intermittent fasting do see problems such as metabolic disturbances, early-onset menopause, and missed periods. In addition, if you find your body experiencing prolonged hormonal issues it could ultimately lead to pale skin, hair loss, acne, decreased energy and the other, similar issues. As long as you don't take your fasting to the extreme, then after the first month or so you should not expect to see any of these issues.

These types of hormonal imbalances are known to occur because women are far more sensitive to signals from their bodies that indicate they are not consuming enough calories on a day to day basis. If enough calories are not being consumed, signals will be sent out and the amount of ghrelin and leptin (two hunger causing hormones) in the body will increase dramatically. The reason that women are so much more susceptible to this issue than men is thanks to the protein known as kisspeptin which occurs in far more quantities in woman than in men. It is used by neurons to decrease the distance between thoughts and actions but is also extremely sensitive to leptin and ghrelin levels.

Metabolism concerns: Your metabolism is intimately tied to your health which means that if you are experiencing physiological or physical challenges, then your health could also be at risk. Luckily, maintaining a healthy diet while exercising, working out and fasting regularly can all help to resolve these types of health challenges. Over time, intermittent fasting has even shown to help balance out hormones which means you just need to be aware of the issue and ride it out while your body adjusts to your new habits.

Protein concerns: Women tend to consume less protein compared to men. It follows, then, that fasting women consume even less protein. Less consumption of protein results in fewer amino acids in the body. Amino acids are essential for the synthesis of insulin-like growth factor in the liver which activates estrogen receptors. The growth factor IGF-1 causes the uterine wall lining to thicken as well as the progression of the reproductive cycle.

A prolonged low protein intake can also affect your estrogen levels, which can also affect your metabolic function and vice versa. This can potentially affect your mood, digestion, cognition, bone formation and more. It can even affect the brain as estrogen is required to stimulate the neurons responsible for ceasing the production of the chemicals that regulate appetite. Essentially, any time your estrogen levels drop noticeably you are likely to end up feeling hungrier than would otherwise be the case.

What to do about it

Crescendo Fasting: As previously discussed, women are naturally more sensitive to feelings of hunger than men are which is why many women find that fasting can be such a challenge. Luckily, there is a variation of intermittent fasting that has been designed to onboard women more easily into an intermittent fasting lifestyle. It is known as Crescendo Fasting and to follow it, all you need to do is start by fasting three days a week on nonconsecutive days.

This approach to fasting tells your body that it is time for the cells to burn fat to obtain energy and to clean house. Crescendo fasting is a game changer for women. It will additionally boost your fertility and help you look and feel your best.

Rules for Crescendo Fasting

1. Fast only 2 or 3 days a week on non-consecutive days. For instance, fast on Tuesdays, Fridays, and Sundays.

2. Fast for 12 to 16 hours only. Do not exceed 16 hours if you can help it.

3. On your fasting days try and do some workouts such as yoga or walking.

4. On other days, do heavier workouts such as skipping or weight training.

5. You are allowed to take lots of water, tea, and coffee as long as they are free of added sugar, sweeteners, or milk.

6. Consider taking 5 – 8 grams of BCAA (branch chain amino acids) on your fast days. They contain very little calories yet provide much-needed fuel to your muscles. These amino acids also take the edge off hunger and fatigue.

You may want to consider having a cup of coffee instead of an 18-hour dry fast. You can add some grass-fed butter and coconut oil. Have this for breakfast but without any protein or carbohydrates. If you feel hungry later on in the day, you can brew another cup. Keep your sugars and fructose levels to a minimum to optimize leptin levels in the body.

If you do not like coffee, you can drink warm water or another beverage to keep your mind off hunger. If you are aged 40 and above or happen to be overweight, then you may want to add grass-fed collagen to your morning cup of coffee on fasting days. Collagen may spike your hunger a little but will definitely reset your leptin which is one of the hunger hormones.

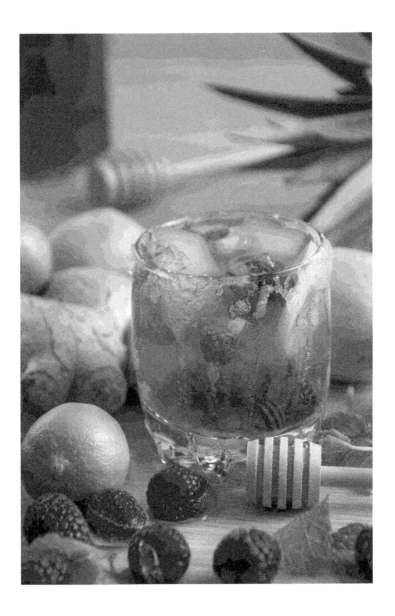

Chapter 5: Intermittent Fasting and Exercise

When it comes to intermittent fasting, it is important to understand how it will affect your ability to exercise if you plan on sticking with the practice in the long-term. The biggest difference you will notice when you are exercising while fasting is that you will naturally feel weaker as less food in your stomach means less available fuel for building new muscles during an exercise routine. As such, if you do plan on exercising regularly while practicing any form of intermittent fasting it is important to take a number of extra precautions in order to ensure your new dietary habits don't end up negatively impacting the effectiveness of your average workout.

Ten muscle biopsies were taken before exercise, as well as three hours after exercise. The results showed that exercising while in a glycogen depleted state was able to increase mitochondrial biogenesis. This is the process by which new mitochondria can form inside the cells. The authors of the study believe that exercising on a low glycogen level diet may be beneficial for improving muscle oxidative capacity.

Exercise and intermittent fasting basics

Regardless if you are looking to improve your strength or your endurance, it is important to keep in mind that fats don't burn as easily as carbs do which means you are going to have less access to immediate energy. On the plus side, however, you will find that you are able to last much longer overall. This is also why you are likely to burn about 20 percent more fat when exercising without carbs in your system than you otherwise would. This is also why you should exercise immediately prior to breaking your fast as opposed to once it has been broken.

Unfortunately, the body doesn't just look for extra fat when it needs energy while exercising, it also requires available protein as well. As protein is stored in your muscles, if you exercise too strenuously then you will actually be hurting your muscles as opposed to helping them. You should be able to get through a moderate exercise routine without risk, however, as long as you don't push it too far. Thus, you should leave the heavier workouts for days when you are consuming more calories on a regular basis.

This means that once your body adapts to its new routine you will naturally have more energy left over for things like exercise in addition to all of your core bodily functions. You can expect it to take about a month for your body to fully adapt to the process. When it comes to merging your existing exercise plan with intermittent fasting, it is vital that you keep in mind that all types of exercise are going to be more difficult right off the bat than what you may remember while your body adjusts to the transition.

This is perfectly natural, of course, you are exercising on an empty stomach after all. Due to the fact that your blood sugar levels and glycogen levels are going to be lower than normal as well, you will likely feel weaker to start to boot. This means it is extremely important to schedule your workout at the appropriate time depending on the goals you have set for yourself. Just make sure you are giving your body the tools it needs to take advantage of all of your hard work.

Exercise tips

What to eat: Sometimes, you will wake up feeling weak instead of ready to start exercising. On these days, you should eat something small before getting started, such as a handful of nuts or a piece of fruit. It's advisable to have a small meal with simple carbs and some protein, such as a protein shake with a banana, or a simple protein bar. If you aren't able to have that much, even a glass of juice can help you make it through your exercise plan more easily in the morning.

If you only have about 30 minutes before your workout, try to pick solid foods that will digest as quickly as possible and limit fiber since it can be rough on your digestive process. If you do decide to work out in a fasted state, always bring some easily digested food just in case. As always, water is extremely important, so make sure you get plenty of that both before, during, and after any physical activity.

Prioritize low-intensity cardio: If you plan on exercising regularly while you are fasting, it is important to limit your cardio to low-intensity options. This means you should still be able to carry on a conversation with relative ease if you are exercising during a fast. Ideally, you are going to want to stick to things like a light jog or 25 minutes on a cardio machine and be sure not to push yourself too hard. It will also be extra important to listen to your body and take a breather if you start to feel dizzy or light-headed which is going to happen much more often than it otherwise would. If you ignore this advice and push your exercise intensity level to the limit then it will make the rest of your workout feel like much more of a struggle regardless of what you are doing.

Choose your battles: This is not to say that you should never push your body to the limit while fasting. Instead, it is important to time your more intense periods of exercise to about an hour after you have eaten. This will give your body time to process the nutrients you have provided for it and will help you to maximize the amount of fat you can lose while still staying properly fueled for the workout by having plenty of glycogen in your system which will also help to reduce the risk of low blood sugar levels. Additionally, if you can afford to alter your fasting schedule slightly, following up a high-intensity workout with a snack that is high in carbs is also encouraged because your muscles will have burned through the available glycogen while still being hungry for more.

Up your protein intake: Standard workout convention suggest that you are going to want to take in between 20 and 30 grams of protein every four hours while you are awake. While intermittent fasting makes this unattainable, you're should still aim to take in between 80 and 120 grams of protein per day. If you are planning a serious strength workout then you should plan to do so between two snacks, if not two full meals.

Exercises to start with while fasting

What follows are a few exercises of the sort you should aim for when exercising while fasting, at least to start. As previously noted, you can certainly take the time to push yourself but starting with exercises like these will get your body used to exercising while fasting without putting you at risk in the process.

Dynamic Stretching: After you have the blood pumping but before you start the workout proper it is important to stretch well to prevent injury.

- Head Circles: Start with your chin facing downwards and rotate your head in a gentle circle in both a clockwise and counterclockwise direction.

- Shoulder Circles: Start with your hand at your sides and slowly roll your shoulders first in one direction and then the other. Ensure your chest and upper back work together.

- Arm Circles: Stretch your arms out and start by making small circles with your arms, gradually expanding until the circumference of the circles extends to include your ears and your hips.

- Torso Circles: Stretch your arms out to the sides and twist your core in one direction and then the other as far as you can without straining yourself.

- Leg Circles: Start by lying on your back with your forearms pressed against the floor. Place one leg straight out and the other bent at the knee while making circles in the air.

Butterflies: For this exercise, you can stand. Bring your hands by your ears so that the elbows are bent, and bend over so that your back is flat. Next, lift the elbows away from the ears, making sure that the shoulder blades are pushing towards one another. Repeat this exercise for at least thirty reps, because of the fact that you will not be using weights. If you want to experience more intensity, using weights for this exercise will certainly intensify the workout.

Kick-ups: To begin this exercise you will want to get on your hands and knees so that your weight is supported by both your knees and your forearms. You will then alternate between legs as you lift one leg off of the ground and kick backwards so your heels face upwards. You will then return the leg to the starting position in one fluid motion. This exercise is beneficial to both the core and the legs.

Hip Bridge: To begin this exercise you will want to lay on your back so that your knees are bent and both of your feet are planted firmly on the floor. You will then want to lift your hips as far off the ground as possible, while at the same time clenching your buttocks, with the end goal being to create a perfectly straight line between your knees as your shoulders. If you are interested in making this exercise even more difficult you can instead aim to keep one foot on the floor while at the same time lifting the other so that it points at the ceiling. This exercise is great for improving hip flexibility while at the same time stretching the spine and improving back strength.

Plank: To begin this exercise you will want to get on your hands and knees before placing all of your weight on your forearms and balancing on your toes. After you are in the position you will then want to tense your entire body, placing special focus on your core, and hold that position for as long as possible. While this might seem simple on the surface, once you try it you will be surprised at just how strenuous it can be. This exercise is useful in strengthening the core.

Superman: To perform this exercise you will want to lay face down on the ground with your arms out in front of you and your legs straight. You will then simply lift both your arms and legs off the ground at the same time, as high as you can. During this exercise you will want to keep your arms and legs stable rather than moving up and down, you will also want to hold for as long as possible. This is a great exercise when it comes to strengthening your back.

Elliptical trainer: Using an elliptical trainer for 45 minutes will burn roughly 330 calories or just shy of three-fourths of what you need to burn in a day to lose 1-2 pounds a week when eating about 1,500 calories per day. This piece of exercise equipment is extremely low impact while still being fairly good at burning calories. If you can find a version that offers an arm as well as leg component, you can burn even more calories at once.

Go for a swim: Swimming at a decent clip for as little as 45 minutes will burn roughly 340 calories or almost 75 percent of what you need to burn in a day to lose 1-2 pounds a week when eating about 1,500 calories per day. Swimming is a great choice for exercising if you have joint issues, are overweight or suffer from arthritis as the water helps minimize pain related to resistance. Start at a slow pace for thirty minutes at a go and work up from there.

Ride a bike: Riding a bike at a decent pace for as little as 45 minutes will burn roughly 380 calories or almost 80 percent of what you need to burn in a day to lose 1-2 pounds a week when eating about 1,500 calories per day. This classic exercise lets you get some fresh air while stretching your muscles and is a great way to ease yourself into an exercise routine. If you plan on riding a bike for exercise it is important to purchase one that is properly fitted to reduce soreness and the chance of injury.

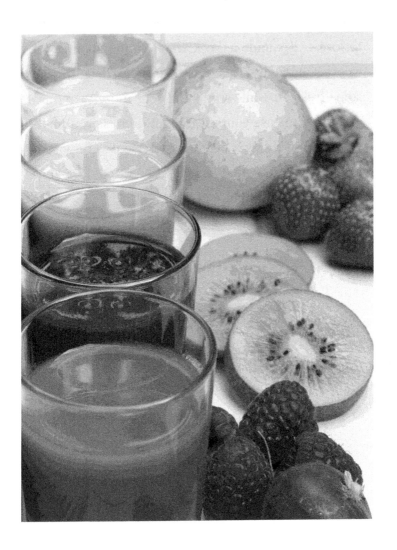

Chapter 6: Intermittent Fasting Tips for Success

Don't make excuses: It is important to not let reasons for not starting an intermittent fast turn into excuses. For example, having a busy schedule or not being able to work in a 12-hour fast are simply reasons that your brain is coming up with to allow you to not try something hard without feeling bad about crying off. The only person who can ensure you are motivated enough to make intermittent fasting work is you, commit to success and follow through on your weight loss goals.

Don't settle for the first plan you try: The shear variety of different intermittent fasting plans available means that, even if you find the first plan you try easy to stick with, there might be a better one out there for you. Not trying multiple plans before you commit can cause you to lose out on something that is even better. After all, if there really isn't anything better out there for you then you can always come back around to your first choice and pick up where you left off. If you don't try them all, you'll never know. Of course, if you don't think you can last the full length of time then there is no point in pushing yourself past your tolerance level, be aware of your limitations and choose accordingly.

Know yourself: Intermittent fasting has a wide variety of proven benefits but it is not for everyone. Before you attempt a fast it is important to have a real dialogue with yourself and consider your level of self-discipline, your current attachment to food, any regular activities that would make fasting difficult or awkward, your general lifestyle and your level of exercise. Deciding to try a different fitness regime is a lot easier on day one than after struggling through a week or more of faulty fasting.

Likewise, while it is important to keep tabs on how your body is responding to intermittent fasting, it is doubly important to monitor your vitals during the initial phase when your body is adjusting to the new feeding times. Some discomfit is to be expected for the first three to four weeks, but anything longer or more severe should be discussed with a doctor as soon as possible.

Don't forget, While your body adjusts to intermittent fasting, there will be times where you are losing weight and times where your body is trying to hold on to every calorie it has. This is natural and to be expected as your body realigns its hormone levels. Every diet is going to have periods of weight loss plateau, that is simply a part of weight loss that cannot be mitigated. As long as you stay consistent weight loss will eventually resume. The worst thing you can do is to try and change things up to get weight loss back on track as that will only make it more difficult for your body to start shedding weight once more.

Use caffeine like a tool: Especially when you first begin training your body to expect food less often, drinking black coffee or a 0 calorie soda every 3 or 4 hours can make it easier to get through the early fasts as caffeine is known to actively suppress the appetite. It is important to not go overboard, however, as many artificial sweeteners have been known to cause health problems when consumed in large amounts. In addition, it is important to not begin to rely on caffeine to the point that your body doesn't actually adapt to the fasting schedule. Feel free to use as much caffeine as you need to get through the first few days of fasting, but keep your intake under control from there as you want your body to be building new habits, not simply have its appetite stunted by caffeine.

Drink plenty of water: While it is easy to see the phrase drink plenty of water and relate it to a command to remain hydrated, what it really means is that while fasting regularly you are going to want to drink a minimum of a gallon of water per day. This practice will not only help you feel full more easily and break your fast early less often, but it will also help your body to continue processing toxins normally during the transition process when it is likely holding on to as much fat as possible.

A gallon of water a day is actually good advice regardless of whether or not you are actively fasting because studies show that nearly forty percent of all adults in the United States are suffering in a mild state of prolonged dehydration. This is especially dangerous for those who are fasting because when left untreated for a prolonged period of time, a severe thirst actually begins to manifest itself as feelings of hunger.

Eat properly: Fasting tends to affect the hormones that regulate hunger such that you won't feel as hungry. This way, you are likely to naturally consume less food than you did previously. You need to be very careful not to consume too few calories during this period because your body will be deprived of essential nutrition. You should eat at least 1200 calories as a minimum. If you do not do this then you will feel extremely hungry the following day and this could affect your ability to perform.

Many people get scared of feeling hungry in the course of the day due to fasting. Yet we all feel hungry at some point during the day even if we consume six meals per day. The problem with this kind of issue is that people often want to eat the minute they feel hungry. The truth is that your body is capable of going without a meal for lengthy periods of time, even 24 hours.

Intermittent fasting is never about what you eat but when you eat. While this is a good mantra to abide with, it sometimes results in problems due to the mindset that fewer meals total allows for more leeway in what is acceptable. Your focus should be more on animal and plant products, both of which should be unprocessed. While this sounds like a paleo diet, it simply refers to having any and all meats and fish. Also, eat foods that grow in the garden such as vegetables, fruits, grains, and pulses and much more. You can consume some processed foods as well. However, try and eat mostly natural foods.

It is important to consume sufficient amounts of fat with your meals. Fat helps prevent the ups and downs of reactive hypoglycemia and sustains your blood sugar. When you do not take enough fat, your insulin goes up, and blood sugar plays up. Then your blood sugar levels drop, and adrenals have to push it back up. This is not a desirable situation at all. Fortunately, good quality, healthy fat can help manage this situation. Coconut or avocado oil are both excellent choices.

Set the right goals: Once you do start your preferred intermittent fasting plan, you are going to want to take into account that a 3,500-calorie deficit is going

Kathleen Moore

to lead to the loss of one pound of fat, but that this equation doesn't take muscle growth into the equation at all. This means that if you are exercising regularly then you may end up losing less weight per week, but still end up looking and feeling better regardless. If you find yourself feeling discouraged based on the results from the scale it is important to consider how long it took you to reach your current weight and fitness level and then give yourself a comparable period of time to get back to where you need to be. Getting to your current point didn't happen overnight and there is no reason to expect changing things up drastically will lead to overnight results either.

Track your progress: Once you begin intermittent fasting, you can start journaling and keeping track of what you are eating. You can easily use your phone as a resource to help you with your intermittent fasting journey. You can use your phone to choose an app that helps with your fasting. A couple of the most popular choices include the Body Fasting app or Fitness Pal. Some apps have extra bonuses you can use, like hiring a personal health coach for extra support.

As you keep track of your journey, do not forget to take note of your victories! Celebrate them. Perhaps you've been fasting three days in a row and are on track perfectly for a week! Celebrate that! On the other hand, if you end up going over on your calorie count one day, that's fine to, as long as you don't use it as an excuse to make additional poor choices as a result. The next day is a new day and you should just get back on track and do not get bogged down if you do not meet your goal. Your journal will also help you see if you are being serious or not. You can trick other people, but you cannot fool yourself.

Get out of the house with some fun distractions: If you are sitting around the house, thinking about food, it is going to be a million times harder to stick with your intermittent fast. There is probably plenty of food around the house, and the more you think about that food, the harder it is to resist the food. And the longer you sit around the house, the harder it will be to resist the temptation to eat, and the more miserable you will be if you don't eat at that time.

The best thing to do is find a way to keep yourself distracted. Get out of the house and go do something.

You can choose to go on a walk. Head to the library and spend some time reading some of your favorite books. Go and spend some time with friends. As long as it keeps you busy and gets you out of the house, it is going to help.

Be aware of the recurring negative thoughts related to food: Often times, a diet fails due to beliefs related to food and eating. Try to become aware of your food beliefs and make an effort to change your mentality. We often think that on special occasions, it is right to let go a bit. There's nothing wrong with eating a little more from time to time, but be honest with yourself about what you consider "special occasions." When events like eating away from home, business lunches, office parties, and other small events all become excuses to let yourself binge, the failure of the diet is just around the corner. Try, therefore, to re-evaluate what occasions can be considered as "special" and when it is better to stick to your original diet plan.

Do you use food as a reward? Many think that after a long busy day, it is normal to deserve to go out for dinner or eat an entire tub of ice cream. Look for alternative ways to reward yourself, which do not include food. For example, take a long hot bath, or go to the movies. There are many ways to reward yourself without using food. Similarly, food is closely linked to numerous rituals. Giving up unhealthy foods may not be easy if you emotionally associate them with certain habits. Make a conscious effort to break these dangerous associations.

Try to be aware of the times you eat too much or make bad food choices, both in terms of food and the things you drink. Whenever you go to the movies, do you buy Coca-Cola and popcorn? Cannot say "no" to a few glasses of wine during the evenings out? Cannot imagine a Saturday morning without coffee and doughnuts? If so, take the extra mile to commit to chopping these associations.

Find ways to reduce your stress: It can be really hard to do a fast when you are feeling a lot of stress. You will have some extra cravings, and if you are dealing with all the stresses in your life, it can be extra difficult to deal with these cravings. While an intermittent fast is not meant to be difficult, it can sometimes be hard to stick with it when you are also dealing with stress.

Since you aren't able to completely get rid of all the stress that you feel in your life, it is better if you learn some effective methods to help you relieve stress when it comes up. You can set up a good exercise routine that helps you to naturally release stress when you feel it coming on. Many people like to practice mindfulness or meditation to get rid of stress. Options like going on a walk, spending time with friends, taking a warm bath, reading a book, and more can help you to reduce your stress so that you can stay on your intermittent fast without worry.

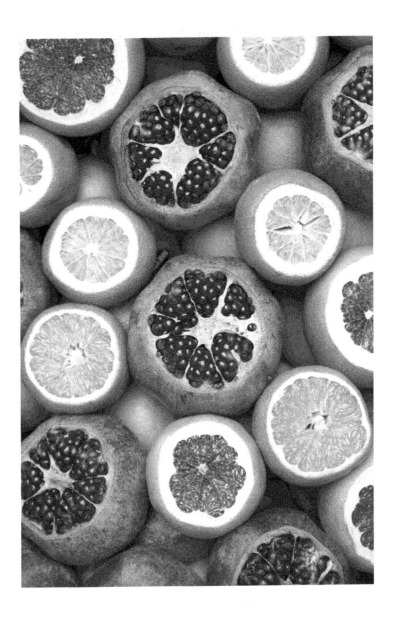

Chapter 7: Intermittent Fasting and the Keto Diet

Many diets today are just fads, but the ketogenic diet has been around for a long time. It may seem like something new that you have come across on the internet, but it was actually developed in the 1920s. At the Mayo Clinic in Minnesota, a doctor named R.M. Wilder was looking for ways to treat patients who suffered from seizures. In his research, he discovered the ketogenic way of eating and used it to treat his patients. During the same era, the ketogenic diet was being pioneered by researchers in pediatric epilepsy at Johns Hopkins in Baltimore. The ketogenic diet proved successful at working miracles for these patients, and it was beloved for a period of time. Eventually, however, anti-seizure medications were introduced to treat patients; and for most people, taking a pill is far easier than completely changing their eating habits. Over time, the ketogenic diet was all but forgotten for decades.

Then, in 1994, Jim Abraham (the Hollywood film director) did an interview about his son Charlie on *Dateline NBC*. Abraham's son Charlie suffered from severe seizures. They had tried many forms of treatment, including all available seizure medications to no avail. When nothing else worked, Abraham sought different answers. In his search to help his son, Abraham rediscovered the ketogenic diet that had been pioneered decades before. The Abraham family started following a ketogenic diet, and soon Charlie was living life seizure-free. Since the ketogenic diet reappeared on the healthy eating scene in the 1990s it has become increasingly popular as people realized just how effective it was at promoting weight loss.

The keto diet is a great fit to pair with intermittent fasting thanks to the fact that they both focus on keeping the amount of insulin in the body as low as possible as a means of promoting weight loss. What makes this pairing especially powerful is that it will essentially allow you to maintain the benefits of your fasted state while eating, as long as you follow a few simple rules.

Before you jump right from starting a fasted state to the keto diet, it is important to understand that you need to give your body the time it needs to respond to one major change at a time. Not only that but if you wait until you have already burned off any excess glucose then making the transition to the keto diet step will be even easier than before. While your body should be ready to go after about 14 days, if you feel as though you are going to need more time then, by all means, take it. Ensuring that these major lifestyle changes sticks are all about doing what feels right for you and adding the keto diet into the mix is no exception. Listening to your body is always guaranteed to produce better results than some by-the-numbers plan.

It is also important to keep in mind that both the keto diet and intermittent fasting are major lifestyle changes which means you don't need to stick to both in a super strict sense unless it works for you. After all, losing weight is not an all or nothing proposition, any forward progress is still worth celebrating.

This is not to say that you should leave the ketogenic state on a whim, however, as willpower does play a big part in being able to intermittently fast successfully. If your willpower isn't quite where you would like it to be then the first thing you should try to do when you feel hungrier than you should is to keep busy. Not only does being bored lead to eating as a way to pass the time, but it also makes the time between now and when you are free to eat again seem to go much more slowly. If you keep a busy schedule during the period of your fast that you are the most hungry you will find that the time almost flies by.

The Keto difference

To understand what makes the keto diet such a natural paring with intermittent fasting, it is useful to understand a little more about how the average diet works. In a conventional/normal diet, you eat foods high in carbohydrates, low in fats, and moderate in proteins. What happens when you eat this type of meal?

When you eat a high carbohydrate meal, your body breaks down the carbohydrates into sugar/glucose. Why does the body do this? The body does this so your body cells can use glucose from the food. It also does this because glucose is your body's main source of energy, which it uses to create ATP, an energy molecule. Once the carbohydrates break down into glucose, the body automatically triggers the production of insulin. Insulin has the following functions:

1. Direct the glucose into your bloodstream.
2. Transport the glucose into your cells and tissues for energy support.
3. Lastly, it supports the storage of excessive glucose not used as energy. The body stores glucose as fat for later use when the body has a low supply of ready energy.

In short, in a conventional diet, your body uses glucose for energy and stores fat as an energy reserve. The main problem with this type of diet is that it stores fat for use in times of hunger, which hardly ever arise because, in the current world, food is readily available. Thus, your chances of using the stored fat are almost zero. This clearly shows you that this type of diet (most conventional diets fall here) is not an ideal way to lose weight. If you are still on the fence, here are a few reasons why you should seriously consider changing your diet.

The first reason why you should abandon this diet is that it encourages fat storage, which translates into weight gain. Secondly, this type of diet stimulates the production of insulin and, as you now know, the work of insulin is to store excess glucose not used as energy. Like reason one, this process encourages fat storage, which leads to weight gain.

The facts above clearly show you are following the wrong diet which means that if you ever hope to see real results you need to change up what exactly it is you are trying to do. The solution, as stated earlier, is to adopt a diet that encourages fat loss rather than fat storage, a Ketogenic diet.

The purpose of the ketogenic diet is to retrain your body to run on better fuel. Rather than glucose, your body will learn to run on fat for fuel. Eating this way will place your body in a position wherein it primarily uses fat, rather than sugar for energy. When your body is burning fat for fuel, it produces molecules called ketones. This is a natural metabolic process of your body called ketosis. Ketosis is achieved by removing most of the sugars and starches in your diet, and instead of following a high healthy fat, moderate protein, low carbohydrate approach to eating.

While ketosis can be brought on by consuming significantly fewer calories than normal, it turns out that cutting out most carbohydrates tricks the body into the same mode. When it comes limiting your carbohydrates, a good guideline to shoot for is to consume less than 15 net carb grams per day. To determine your net carbs, you simply add up how many carbohydrates you consumed in a 24-hour period and then subtract that number from the amount of fiber you consumed during that same amount of time.

Prior to making any major dietary changes, you should always consult a healthcare professional or registered nutritionist to ensure that you aren't accidentally doing more harm to yourself then good. When it comes to sticking to the ketogenic diet, net carbohydrates should only make up 5 percent of your diet, 25 percent should be protein and the remaining

70 percent should be made up of healthy fats. Wheats and starches of all types should be off limits and most carbohydrates should come from nuts, vegetables, and dairy product.

Dark, leafy green vegetables should be a staple of most meals as should several natural fats and a good source of protein. Consider meals such as olive oil coated chicken with vegetables or roasted cauliflower with steak slathered in butter. If you need to snack, reach for healthy, fatty options such as seeds, nuts, peanut butter or cheeses. Despite the fact that fats have received a bad rap in the media, without carbohydrates holding you back, you will find that they are far more useful than you have been led to believe.

Additional benefits

While literally helping to melt the fat off of your body is nice, the keto diet actually offers numerous other benefits that run the gamut from being weight loss related to helping to potentially save your life. Remember, the following benefits only remain in effect while you are in ketosis and the longer the state persists the more potent the results will be.

Appetite reduction: In addition to reducing existing fat, the ketogenic diet is also well-known for its ability to reduce hunger overall, making it less likely that you will eat past the point of feeling full, naturally keeping you trim without having to resort to counting calories. Even when you are transitioning to the keto diet, during the period when cravings and unwarranted feelings of hunger are at their most aggressive, you will find that the foods described in later chapters really do help you to feel more full for a greater period of time.

This is the case due to a natural byproduct of the ketone creation process as, in their natural state, ketones produce a hormone known as cholecystokinin which combats the hunger causing hormone ghrelin. Typically, this hormone is produced as a result of food moving through your intestines, but while in a state of ketosis you will find that it is constantly being pumped into your system, making you less hungry all the time as a result. In fact, the *American Journal of Clinical Nutrition* found that during a recent clinical trial that the hormone production never decreased in a full 8-week study while ketosis was in process before returning to original levels within just 7 days after the state of ketosis was concluded.

Combat serious disease: In addition to making you thinner and making you wonder less about when your next meal is going to hurry up and arrive, the keto diet can actually directly reduce your risk of several types of cancer as these cancer cells are known to feed on glucose just like regular cells do. These types of cancers find it difficult to survive purely on ketones which means they will grow far more slowly than would otherwise be the case if your body is relying on fat as its main source of fuel. What's more, because the keto diet is more in line with the type of nutrition the human body is built to process, it makes it easier for core processes to take place which makes it a natural choice for combating both dementia and Alzheimer's disease.

This is thanks to the fact that the neurons in your brain are designed to get their energy from glucose, however, this is very much the case of too much of a good thing being in effect. This is because if the brain receives too many carbohydrates over a prolonged period of time it can become more resistant to insulin. This, in turn, will ultimately cause it to work harder to generate the same results. Luckily, the brain can function on ketones as a byproduct of the process works for glucose specific processes in a pinch. What's more, it can do so indefinitely without having to worry about any of the other issues that might otherwise be the case.

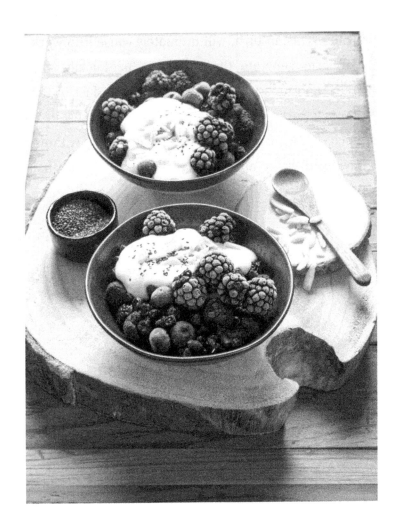

Chapter 8: Transitioning to the Keto Diet

This section is going to show you how to adopt the ketogenic diet and lose excess body fat and weight in an easy and natural way. If that sounds good, stop wasting time and get started right away:

As a beginner, your main goal and the reason behind adopting this diet is to reach the metabolic state of ketosis. To reach that state, you must consider two factors.

1.   What you are eating

2.   The quantity of the food nutrients you are eating.

The two factors above are very important because they will determine whether you will reach the metabolic state of ketosis and how fast you get there.

Dealing with the keto flu

Despite the healthy advantages of switching to the ketogenic diet, making the transition will cause your body to react negatively at first as you are taking away its primary energy source. Thanks to the high amount of carbohydrates previously found in your diet for years, your body has plenty of options for breaking down carbohydrates, but relatively few on deck to turn fat into energy. As such, it will initially take your body longer to break down this new energy sources which will cause you to feel under the weather until your body gets with the program.

During the first week or two of your transition into the ketogenic lifestyle, you are going to experience a range of flu-like symptoms as your body stops using glucose for fuel and switches to ketones instead. First, you will feel sluggish and tired, because your body literally doesn't have any fuel powering its core systems. This is because you have allowed your body to become extremely efficient when it comes to breaking down glucose, while at the same time never giving it the opportunity to develop the tools it needs to break down fats as effectively. What this means is that until it connects all the dots you are going to feel like you are running on empty, but only because you are.

Additionally, you are going to likely feel as though you have a cold, aches, chills, the whole nine yards. What you are actually going to be experiencing is withdrawal, the same as you would when removing any other harmful and addictive substance from your diet. It will all ultimately be worth it, however, as once your body gets with the new program you will be on your way to living the keto lifestyle in perpetuity.

When you first start trying to adapt to a ketogenic lifestyle, if you are afraid that your carb withdrawal is going to be extremely severe, then you may instead want to start out by slowly cutting out the carbs from your regular diet. There is nothing that says you need to jump directly from eating a diet that is likely 60 percent carbs to a diet that is less than 15 net carbs per day, cutting down slowly can make the final transition far more manageable.

While it may seem as though your body is rejecting your new intended dietary habits, it is important to remember that this is simply part of the process if you are interested in putting your body into a long-term state of ketosis. Having a firm idea of what's in store will likely also make it easier to manage the transition, remember, forewarned is forearmed. Stick with it and you will soon feel better than you ever thought possible.

It is important to not try and mitigate the symptoms by eating more than 15 net grams of carbohydrates per day, this will only prolong the transition symptoms, not make them easier to manage. What's more, you won't be in true ketosis as that requires a stricter limit, essentially you will be making yourself feel worse for no measurable gain. The sooner the transition period ends; the sooner you can start maximizing your weight loss potential.

Know Your Macros

The name macros stands for macronutrients, the three nutrients you usually consume during your meals. These three main macronutrients are fats, carbohydrates, and proteins. To enter ketosis, you will first need to know how you can balance these three nutrients in your meals. Below is how each of these three nutrients affects ketosis:

Fats are normally 90 percent ketogenic and 10 percent anti-ketogenic because the glycerol present in fats produces a small amount of oxygen. Proteins are 45 percent ketogenic and 58 percent anti-ketogenic because the body turns half of the proteins you ingest into glucose. Carbohydrates are 100 percent anti-ketogenic because they raise the level of insulin and blood glucose.

As you can see, fats have the highest ketogenic percentage followed by proteins and then carbohydrates that have a zero ketogenic percentage. Therefore, to enter ketosis, your food needs a lot of fats, a reasonable amount of proteins, and few if any carbohydrates.

Protein: If only 25 percent of what you eat in a day can be protein then it is important to give that protein extra consideration. First and foremost, it is important to keep in mind that not all proteins are good for you, specifically those that are not of an organic nature as they are likely to contain high amounts of both bacteria and steroids. As such, you should always take special care to choose to only eat animal protein that is both grass fed and organic. The following are all acceptable protein choices, as long as you stick fast to the 25 percent per day rule.

Fats and oils: First and foremost, when it comes to balancing out the fats that you consume each day it is important to balance your intake of omega 3 and omega 6 as you need a balance of both to maintain a healthy lifestyle in the long term. Fish contain plenty of both types of omega fat, though if you are not a fan of fish then fish oil supplements can work just as well.

When it comes to the best monounsaturated or saturated fats the best choices are those that are the most chemically stable as this is a sign that they are good for your health as well. Great choices in this category include things like avocado oil, egg yolks, coconut oil, organic, grass-fed butter and macadamia nuts in moderation.

Carbohydrates: With only a very small percentage of your overall daily intake dedicated to carbohydrates, it is important that you make the amount you can eat as effective as possible. The best way to do this is to focus on vegetables that have the overall lowest amount of carbohydrates as possible so you can maximize the nutritional impact of that portion of your diet. The vegetables that you should avoid at all costs include peppers of all colors, carrots, tomatoes, corn, squash, and peas.

On the other hand, the vegetables that you are going to want to stock up on because they have the least amount of carbs overall include things like kale, garlic, sprouts, cabbage, shallots, spinach, radishes, olives, leeks, cucumbers, cauliflower, asparagus, chives, broccoli, bok choy and dill pickles. If you are curious about a vegetable that isn't on this list, all you need to do is ask yourself if it is green, sweet or starchy. If it isn't any of these then you are in the clear.

Dairy: When working towards ketosis for the first time you are going to want to limit your dairy as much as possible as it is virtually guaranteed to cause your insulin levels to spike. Furthermore, dairy contains both casein and whey which can skew your daily protein average which means it can definitely skew your macros if you aren't careful. While during the initial transition you will want to avoid all dairy, after that you can then include unsweetened milk, mascarpone cheese, whipping cream, sour cream, cottage cheese, and cream cheese. For other cheeses, either hard or soft, you will want to remember that 1 gram of cheese typically contains 1 carb.

Sugar substitutes: After you have reached ketosis for the first time it is important to keep your sugar consumption in mind as it will directly reflect the amount of insulin that is in your system at a given time. It is also important to be quite choosey when it comes to artificial sweeteners as both dextrose and maltodextrin will make staying in a ketogenic state more difficult than it really needs to be. Artificial sweeteners to use include nectar from the agave plant, erythritol, stevia, sucralose, xylitol, and monk fruit.

Spices: One area of the kitchen that contains more carbohydrates than you might expect is the spice rack. While normally it isn't enough to warrant being part of the discussion, if you can only spare five percent of your daily total, every little bit counts. The seasoning choices to prioritize include sea salt, but black pepper, cayenne pepper, basil, cinnamon, chili powder, cilantro, turmeric, cumin, parsley, sage, oregano, rosemary, and thyme as long as they are not used to excess.

Getting started tips for success

Monitor your progress: When it comes to ensuring your time spent on the ketogenic diet is as fruitful as possible it is important to work to fine tune your ketosis level which means you will need to purchase what is known as a blood meter to check your ketone levels. Ideally, you will want your ketone levels to be at anywhere from 3 and .5 millimolars to maximize your weight loss goals.

If, after testing yourself you find that your ketone level is still less than .5 millimolars then your body is not yet in a state of full ketosis which means you might want to cut your carbohydrates slightly more than what is outlined below. If you are somewhere between 1.5 ketones and .5 ketones, then your body is in the early stages of ketosis which is right where you want to be during weeks 1 and 2. If your ketone number ever rises above 3, however, then this is a sign that you are not consuming enough calories in a day, which can be an issue for those who exercise during week 3. Either add in an extra recipe from the side dish chapter or exercise less to get your ketone level back to where it should be.

Jump in with both feet: Yes, it has been said before but really, really, really, stop eating low fat options. Throw out anything with low fat on the label, buy whole milk, flood your vegetables with butter, leave the skin on the chicken and fry all the things that can be fried. 70 percent of your diet needs to be fat, without it, you won't see the results you are looking for.

Monitor your electrolytes properly: While in ketosis you will burn through electrolytes like no one's business. It is important to have a replacement plan in place before you start and stick to it religiously. Consider coconut water, bone broth or sugar-free Gatorade for starters. It doesn't matter what you choose, just that you stick to it regularly. Failure to do so will lead to an onset of flu-like symptoms.

Avoid fruit and beer: Fruit contains 10 percent sugar by weight as well as a surprising number of carbohydrates. This sugar can slow down the rate at which your body burns fat as the sugar will get burned off first instead. Fruit is nature's candy and like all candy should be consumed in moderation.

Much like fruit, beer is high in carbohydrates and many are surprisingly high in sugar as well. Beer is literally liquid bread and should be avoided as such. When it comes to consuming alcoholic beverages, stick to dry white or red wine, vodka or cognac. If you are looking for a cocktail, go with lime, soda, and vodka instead of a highly sweetened cocktail.

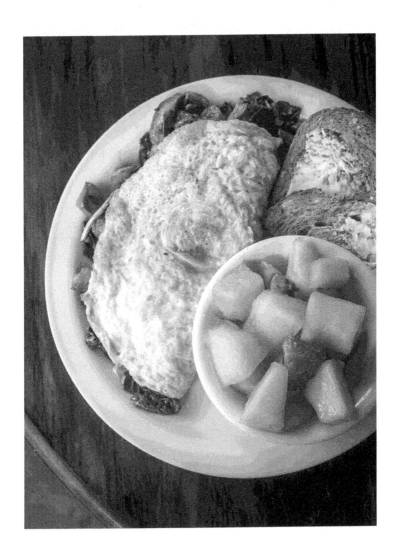

Chapter 9: Keto Diet Recipes

Breakfast recipes

Coconut granola bars

Total preparation time (including cooking): 3 hours
Yields: 8 servings

Nutrition Stats (one serving)
- Net Carbs .7 g
- Fats: 2.7 g
- Calories: 102
- Protein: 14.2 g

What to Use
- Flax eggs (2)
- Medjool dates (4 chopped)
- Sea salt (.5 tsp.)
- Baking powder (.5 tsp.)
- Chia seeds (2 T)
- Vanilla beans (2 tsp. ground)

- Coconut (.25 c shredded)
- Flax meal (.25 c)
- Coconut butter (.5 c)
- Maple syrup (.5 c)
- Rolled oats (1.5 c gluten free)

What to Do

- Add the oats, flax meal, shredded coconut, ground vanilla beans, and baking powder together in a small bowl and combine thoroughly.
- Separately, combine the maple syrup, dates and flax eggs in another bowl.
- Mix the two bowls together and combine thoroughly.
- Grease the slow cooker and line it with parchment paper.
- Add in the ingredients to the slow cooker and pat it down well, take care to make sure it is distributed evenly. Adjust the slow cooker temperature to low and leave it be, covered for about 2.5 hours. You will know it is done when the middle ceases to be mushy.

- After the bars have finished cooking, remove them by gently pulling out the parchment paper.
- Let the results cool 40 minutes before cutting them into bars.

Aprium and avocado smoothie

Total preparation time (including cooking): 5 minutes
Yields: 1 serving

Nutrition Stats (one serving)
Net Carbs: 6.5 grams
Protein: 24 grams
Fats: 24 grams
Calories: 512

What to Use
- Ice cubes (6)
- Your choice of sweetener (to taste)
- Avocado (.5 medium)
- Plain whey protein powder (1 scoop)
- Coconut oil (2 T)

- Lime (.5 juiced)
- Aprium (1 pitted)
- Collard greens (1 oz.)
- Almonds (3 T)

What to Do

- Slice the avocado lengthwise before removing the seeds and the skin. Add the sliced avocado, along with the remaining ingredients to your blender.
- Add all of the ingredients, save the ice cubes, to the blender and blend on a low speed until pureed. Thin with water as needed.
- Add in the ice cubes and blend until the smoothie reaches your desired consistency.

Lunch recipes

Asian Mason Jar Salad

Total preparation time (including cooking): 25 minutes

Yields: 4 servings

Nutrition Stats (one serving)

- Protein: 28 grams

- Net Carbs: 5.4 grams

- Fats: 23 grams

- Calories: 524

What to Use - Salad

- Snap peas (1.3 c halved)

- Cucumber ((1.3 c sliced)

- Carrots ((1.3 c grated)

- Unsalted cashews (1 c)

- Red pepper (1 julienned)

- Baby spinach (2 c sliced)

- Napa cabbage (2 c sliced)

- Rotisserie chicken (2 c shredded)

- Green onions (2 T sliced)

What to Use - Dressing

- Garlic clove (1 minced)

- Honey (1 T)

- Ginger (1 T minced)

- Olive oil (1 T)

- Sesame seeds (1 tsp.)

- Sriracha sauce (1 tsp.)

- Toasted sesame oil (2.5 T)

- Cilantro (2 T)
- Rice vinegar (2 T)
- Low-sodium soy sauce (3 T)

What to Do
- Whisk sesame seeds, honey, cilantro, garlic, ginger, sriracha, olive oil, toasted sesame oil, vinegar, and soy sauce together.
- Toss spinach and Napa cabbage together.
- Assemble jars by add three T of dressing, .3 C snap peas, .25 C chicken, .25 C cashews, and a sprinkle of green onion. Serve now or place in the fridge.

Spicy Thai Chicken

Total preparation time (including cooking): 15 minutes
Yields: 4 servings

Nutrition Stats (one serving)
- Protein: 25 grams
- Net Carbs: 5.1 grams
- Fats: 31.6 grams
- Calories: 298

What to Use

- Coconut oil (2 T)
- Pepper (as desired)
- Salt (as desired)
- Basil (3 T chopped)
- Hoisin sauce (.25 c)
- Coleslaw mix (.25 c)
- Green onions (.5 chopped)
- Red bell pepper (.25 sliced thin)
- Garlic (4 cloves minced)
- Ginger (1 T minced)
- Red curry paste (2 T)
- Chicken (1 lb. ground)

What to Do

- Add the coconut oil to a skillet before placing it on the stove over a burner turned to a high heat. Add in the chicken and let it brown before breaking it up with the help of a wooden spoon.
- Mix in the red curry paste, coleslaw, peppers, and garlic and let everything cook for 3 minutes before adding in the

green onions and hoisin sauce and tossing well.

- Remove the skillet from the burner, add the basil and toss.

Asparagus and Lemon Chicken

Total preparation time (including cooking): 30 minutes

Yields: 4 servings

Nutrition Stats (one serving)
- Protein: 12 grams
- Net Carbs: 5 grams
- Fats: 18.7 grams
- Calories: 183

What to Use
- Coconut oil (2 T divided)
- Pepper (as desired)
- Salt (as desired)
- Chicken stock (1 c)
- Dijon mustard (1 T)
- Lemon zest (.5 lemon)

- Lemon juice (3 T)
- Garlic (2 cloves crushed)
- Asparagus stalks (1 lb.)
- Tapioca flour (.25 c)
- Chicken breast (4 skinless, boneless)

What to Do

- Start by placing each of the chicken breasts between a pair of pieces of plastic wrap before pounding them down until they are about .25 inches thick each.
- Add the pepper, salt, and flour to a mixing bowl before adding in the chicken and ensuring it is well coated.
- Add 1 T of the oil to a skillet before placing it on top of a burner turned to a high/medium heat. Once the oil is thoroughly heated, add in the chicken and let it cook approximately 5 minutes per side or until it reaches an internal temperature of at least 165 degrees. Remove it from the skillet while you cook the asparagus.

- Add the rest of the oil to the skillet before adding in the asparagus stalks and letting them cook for 60 seconds before adding in the garlic and letting it cook for yet another minute.
- While it is cooking, mix together the mustard and lemon juice in a small c and whisk well. Add the results to the skill and turn the heat up to allow the liquid to boil.
- Once it does so, reduce the heat and allow it to boil for approximately 3 minutes until the asparagus becomes tender.
- Plate the chicken and top with the asparagus and the excess liquid.

Mini Keto Tacos

Total preparation time (including cooking): 45 minutes
Yields: 11 servings

Nutrition Stats (one serving)
- Protein: 13.1 grams
- Net Carbs: 1.7 grams
- Fats: 19.4 grams

- Calories: 241

What to Use-Shell

- Water (2 T chilled)
- Cayenne Pepper (.25 tsp.)
- Paprika (.25 tsp.)
- Oregano (1 tsp.)
- Xanthan Gum (1 tsp.)
- Salt (.25 tsp.)
- Butter (5 T)
- Coconut Flour (3 T)
- Almond   Flour   (1   c   blanched)

What to Use-Filling

- Cinnamon (.25 tsp.)
- Worcestershire sauce (1 tsp.)
- Salt (1 tsp.)
- Pepper (.5 tsp.)
- Cumin (1 tsp.)
- Garlic (2 tsp.)
- Yellow mustard (2 tsp.)
- Olive oil (1 T)
- Tomato paste (2 T)
- Spring onion (3 stalks)
- Mushrooms (3 oz.)

- Beef (14 oz. ground)
- Cheddar cheese (.3 c)

What to Do

- Start by making sure your oven is heated to 325F.
- Add the shell ingredients cayenne pepper, paprika, oregano, salt, coconut flour, and blanched almond flour to a food processor before adding in the butter and pulse until the results form a crumble.
- Add in 1 T chilled water and pulse until the dough is malleable.
- Add the results to the freezer and let them cool for 10 minutes.
- Roll out the dough as desired before using a cookie cutter to cut out sections of the dough.
- Add the results to a whoopee pan.
- Coat a pan in the oil and place it on the stove above a burner that has been turned to a high/medium heat.
- Add the onions and garlic to the pan and let them sauté, you will be able to tell when they are finished because they will be practically see through.

- Mix in the ground beef and let it sear prior to seasoning with the salt, pepper, garlic, cumin and Worcestershire sauce.
- Add in the mushrooms and mix well before adding in the mustard and tomato paste.
- Add the results to the shells before topping with the cheese and placing the whoopee pan in the oven for 20 minutes to bake before letting it broil for an additional 5 minutes.
- Let the mini tacos cool completely, prior to eating.

Dinner recipes

Zucchini Ravioli

Total preparation time (including cooking): 50 minutes
Yields: 8 servings

Nutrition Stats (one serving)
- Protein: 32.8 grams
- Net Carbs: 4.6 grams
- Fats: 37 grams
- Calories: 365

What to Use

- Extra-virgin olive oil (2 T)
- Zucchini (4)
- Ricotta (2 c)
- Parmesan (.5 c grated fine)
- Egg (1 large, beaten lightly)
- Basil (.25 c torn, divided)
- Garlic (1 clove minced)
- Salt (as desired)
- Pepper (as desired)
- Marinara sauce (.5 c)
- Mozzarella (.5 c shredded)

What to Do

- Ensure your oven is heated to 375F.
- Prepare a baking dish by greasing it using olive oil.
- Add 2 T basil, the parmesan cheese, and ricotta cheese the ricotta cheese to a mixing bowl before seasoning as desired.
- Lay a pair of zoodles out so that they overlap horizontally and then two more that cross the first pair so that the results for a "T".

- Add 1 T of the parmesan mixture to the center of the zucchini T. Fold the zoodle strips together so that they cover the middle and form a solid square. Flip the resulting ravioli over and place it into the baking dish with the folds facing down. Repeat as needed.
- Once all of the ravioli have been placed in the baking sheet top with the marinara sauce and additional mozzarella cheese.
- Place the baking dish in the oven for about 25 minutes and top with additional parmesan prior to serving.

Tuna Panini

Total preparation time (including cooking): 25 minutes
Yields: 4 servings

Nutrition Stats (one serving)
- Protein: 31 grams
- Net Carbs: 4.1 grams
- Fats: 26 grams
- Calories: 572

What to Use

- Extra-virgin olive oil (2 tsp.)
- Salt (as desired)
- Black pepper (as desired)
- Wholegrain bread (8 slices)
- Lemon juice (1 tsp.)
- Capers (1 tsp. chopped)
- Kalamata olives (1 T chopped, pitted)
- Red onion (2 T minced)
- Artichoke hearts (2 T chopped)
- Feta cheese (.25 c crumbled)
- Plum tomato (1 chopped)
- Light tuna (12 oz. chunked)

What to Do

- Flake the tuna in a bowl with the help of a fork. Mix in the pepper, salt, lemon juice, capers, olives, onion, artichokes, feta, and tomato and combine well.
- Place .5 c of the tuna mixture on half of the slices. And top the sandwiches.
- Add the oil to a skillet and place the skillet on the stove over a burner set to a high/medium heat. Add 2 panni to the skillet at a time, and cook the first side for 2 minutes, reduce the

heat to low/medium and cook the other side for 2 minutes.

- Add additional oil for the second set of sandwiches as needed.

Beef Chili

This recipe makes 12 servings and requires about 45 minutes of preparation and 6 hours of cooking on a low heat.

Nutrition Stats (one serving)
- Fiber 2 g
- Carbohydrates (in total): 8 g
- Fats: 8 g
- Calories: 217
- Protein: 26 g

What to Use
- Salt (as needed)
- Pepper (as needed)
- Chicken broth (2.5 c)
- Green chilis (4 oz.)
- Chili powder (.5 tsp.)

- Paprika (.5 tsp.)
- Cumin (1 T)
- Oregano 91 tsp.)
- Garlic (5 cloves chopped)
- Yellow onion (2 chunked)
- Pork roast (3 lbs. cubed)
- Extra virgin olive oil (2 T)
- Anaheim peppers (2)
- Tomatillos (2 lbs. de-husked)

What to Do

- Ensure your oven is heated to 450F. Cover a baking sheet with tin foil and set the tomatillos and the Anaheim pepper onto it and then place the sheet on the oven's top rack. Let them roast for 25 minutes until the tops have charred.
- While they are cooking, add the olive oil to a frying pan and place it top of the stove over a burner turned to a high heat. Add in the pork and let it brown on all sides which should take about 5 minutes. Once it has browned, add it to the slow cooker.

- Turn the heat on the burner to medium/high before adding in the onion and letting it cook about 2 minutes. Mix in the seasoning, paprika, cumin and garlic and let everything cook another minute before adding in the chicken broth. Let the pan simmer before adding it to the slow cooker.

- Remove the charred skin after the tomatillos and peppers have finished cooking before adding them to a blender with the green chilis and cilantro. Blend well.

- Pour the results into your slow cooker. Adjust the slow cooker temperature to low and leave it be, covered, for 6 hours.

Keto Carnitas

Total preparation time (including cooking): 8 hours and 15 minutes

Yields: 6 servings

Nutrition Stats (one serving)

- Protein: 8 grams
- Net Carbs: 0grams
- Fats: 19 grams

- Calories: 265

What to Use

- Water (1 c)
- Pepper (as desired)
- Salt (as desired)
- Garlic (4 T minced)
- Chili powder (2 T)
- Thyme (2 T)
- Cumin (2 T)
- Onion (1 large)
- Bacon grease (2 T)
- Pork butt (8 lbs.)

What to Do

- Rub the pork with the seasonings before adding it to the slow cooker.
- Add in the remaining ingredients before letting the slow cooker cook, covered for about 8 hours.

Mini Keto Tacos

Total preparation time (including cooking): 45 minutes

Yields: 5 servings

Nutrition Stats (one serving)

- Protein: 13.1 grams
- Net Carbs: 1.7 grams
- Fats: 29.4 grams
- Calories: 241

What to Use - Shell

- Water (2 T chilled)
- Cayenne Pepper (.25 tsp.)
- Paprika (.25 tsp.)
- Oregano (1 tsp.)
- Xanthan Gum (1 tsp.)
- Salt (.25 tsp.)
- Butter (5 T)
- Coconut Flour (3 T)
- Almond Flour (1 c blanched)

What to Use - Filling

- Cinnamon (.25 tsp.)
- Worcestershire sauce (1 tsp.)
- Salt (1 tsp.)
- Pepper (.5 tsp.)

- Cumin (1 tsp.)
- Garlic (2 tsp.)
- Yellow mustard (2 tsp.)
- Olive oil (1 T)
- Tomato paste (2 T)
- Spring onion (3 stalks)
- Mushrooms (3 oz.)
- Beef (14 oz. ground)
- Cheddar cheese (.3 c)

What to Do

- Start by making sure your oven is heated to 325F.
- Add the shell ingredients cayenne pepper, paprika, oregano, salt, coconut flour, and blanched almond flour to a food processor before adding in the butter and pulse until the results form a crumble.
- Add in 1 T chilled water and pulse until the dough is malleable.
- Add the results to the freezer and let them cool for 10 minutes.
- Roll out the dough as desired before using a cookie cutter to cut out sections of the dough.

- Add the results to a whoopee pan.
- Coat a pan in the oil and place it on the stove above a burner that has been turned to a high/medium heat.
- Add the onions and garlic to the pan and let them sauté, you will be able to tell when they are finished because they will be practically see through.
- Mix in the ground beef prior to seasoning with the salt, pepper, garlic, cumin and Worcestershire sauce.
- Add in the mushrooms and mix well before adding in the mustard and tomato paste.
- Place the whoopee pan in the oven for 20 minutes to bake
- Add the beef mixture to the shells before topping with the cheese and letting it broil for an additional 5 minutes.
- Let the mini tacos cool completely, prior to eating.

Snack recipes

Olive and tomato fat bomb

Total preparation time (including cooking): 45 minutes

Yields: 5 servings

Nutrition Stats (one serving)

- Protein: 3.7 grams
- Net Carbs: 1.7 grams
- Fats: 17.1 grams
- Calories: 164

What to Use

- Parmesan cheese (5 T grated)
- Salt (.25 tsp.)
- Black pepper (as desired)
- Garlic (2 cloves crushed)
- Kalamata olives (4 pitted)
- Sun-dried tomatoes (4 pieces drained)
- Oregano (2 T chopped)
- Thyme (2 T chopped)
- Basil (2 T chopped)
- Butter (.25 c)

- Cream cheese (.5 c)

What to Do

- Chop the butter and add it to a small mixing bowl with the cream cheese and leave them both to soften for about 30 minutes. Mash together and mix well to combine.
- Add in the Kalamata olives and sun-dried tomatoes and mix well before adding in the herbs and seasonings. Combine thoroughly before placing the mixing bowl in the refrigerator to allow the results to solidify.
- Once it has solidified, form the mixture into a total of 5 balls using an ice cream scoop. Roll each of the finished balls into the parmesan cheese before plating.
- Extras can be stored in the refrigerator in an air-tight container for up to 7 days.

Cauliflower Fritters

Total preparation time (including cooking): 35 minutes

Yields: 6 servings

Nutrition Stats (one serving)

- Protein: 3.2 grams
- Net Carbs: .8 grams
- Fats: 15.7 grams
- Calories: 147

What to Use

- Lemon pepper (1.5 tsp)
- Eggs (3 large)
- Onion (3 oz. chopped)
- Baking powder (.5 tsp)
- Parmesan cheese (.5 c grated)
- Almond flour (.5 c)
- Salt (1 tsp.)
- Cauliflower (1 lb.)

What to Do

- Grate cauliflower in a food processor. Place in a bowl, sprinkle with salt. Let sit for 10 minutes.
- Place chopped onions in a bowl. Squeeze all the water out of cauliflower and put it with the onion. Add almond flour, baking powder,

seasonings, and cheese. Combine. Mix in three eggs and mix again.

- Skillet Method: Heat frying pan and 1 T oil. Put .25 c batter into hot skillet. Pat down with a spatula to make a pancake. Cook about three minutes on each side. Drain on paper towels. Do not flip until the bottom is well browned.
- Oven Method: Your oven should be at 400F. Place foil on two baking sheets. Put .25 c batter at a time on the baking sheet. Shape into either circles or rectangles. Bake about 12 minutes. Turn them over and bake for 12 more minutes.
- Store any leftovers in the fridge. Reheat in a dry skillet to make them crispy again.

Fishy fat bomb

Total preparation time (including cooking): 70 minutes
Yields: 6 servings

Nutrition Stats (one serving)
- Protein: 3.2 grams
- Net Carbs: 0.8 grams
- Fats: 15.7 grams

- Calories: 147

What to Use
- Salt (1 pinch)
- Dill (2 T chopped)
- Lemon juice (1 T)
- Smoked salmon (1.8 oz.)
- Ghee (.3 c)
- Cream cheese (.5 c)

What to Do
- Add the smoked salmon, butter and cream cheese to a food processor along with the dill and lemon juice and pulse generously.
- Prepare a serving tray by covering it with parchment paper before spooning out the salmon mixture in 2.5 T dollops.
- Top with additional dill and let chill in the refrigerator for at least 60 minutes prior to serving.

Dessert recipes

Cinnamon and Coconut Bites

Total preparation time (including cooking): 95 minutes

Yields: 12 servings

Nutrition Stats (one serving)

- Protein: 17.6 grams
- Net Carbs: 2.2 grams
- Fats: 24.5 grams
- Calories: 367

What to Use

- Coconut shreds (1 c)
- Stevia powder extract (1 tsp.)
- Cinnamon (.5 tsp.)
- Nutmeg (.5 tsp.)
- Vanilla extract (1 tsp.)
- Coconut milk (1 c)
- Coconut butter (1 c)

What to Do

- Place a glass bowl on top of a sauce pan which contains 2 inches of water for the purpose of making a double boiler.

- Add the coconut butter, coconut milk, vanilla extract, nutmeg, cinnamon and stevia powder to the double boiler and place the double boiler on the stove over a burner turned to a medium heat.

- Mix the ingredients well as they melt.

- Once the ingredients are well combined, remove the bowl from the top of the pan and set it in the refrigerator to cool for 30 minutes.

- Roll the contents of the bowl into balls that are approximately one inch in diameter and then roll them in the shredded coconut to coat.

- Refrigerate for an additional hour prior to serving.

Nougat Treats

Total preparation time (including cooking): 30 minutes

Yields: 40 servings

Nutrition stats (one serving)
- Protein: 1.2 grams
- Net Carbs: 0.2 grams
- Fats: 26 grams
- Calories: 76

What to Use
- Vanilla (1 tsp)
- Cocoa powder (1 T)
- Peanut butter (8 T)
- Coconut milk (14 oz.)
- Coconut oil (.5 c divided)
- Dark chocolate (7.5 oz)

What to Do
- Melt half of the chocolate and mix in two T of the coconut oil.
- Pour this into a parchment-lined a greased square baking dish, and place in the fridge to harden.
- Add the solid part of the coconut milk to a pot and allow it to come to a simmer.

- Add in .25 c coconut oil, vanilla, cocoa powder, and nut butter. Mix together until smooth. If it starts to split, use an electric mixer to bring it together.
- Take the mixture off the heat and pour into the baking dish. Refrigerate again until firm. Melt the rest of the chocolate just like in step one.
- Spread this over top of the chilled nougat and refrigerate again.
- Slice into 40 pieces and keep in a storage container in the fridge.

Granola

Total preparation time (including cooking): 40 minutes
Yields: 12 servings

Nutrition stats (one serving)
- Protein: 7.9 grams
- Net Carbs: 0.4 grams
- Fats: 31.6 grams
- Calories: 337

What to Use

- Swerve (.5c)
- Salt (1 tsp.)
- Pumpkin seeds (1 c)
- Raw almonds (.5c)
- Raw walnuts (.5c)
- Vanilla extract (1 tsp.)
- Raw pecans (.5c)
- Raw hazelnuts (.5c)
- Raw sunflower seeds (1 c)
- Vanilla Stevia (1 tsp)
- Ground cinnamon (1 tsp)
- Unsweetened shredded coconut (1 c)
- Coconut oil (.3 c)

What to Do

- Set the cooker to sauté then add the coconut oil and melt. When melted, add the vanilla extract and Stevia. Stir well before adding coconut, seeds, and nuts. Stir mixture well to coat all ingredients.
- In bowl whisk salt, cinnamon, and swerve then sprinkle with seeds and nuts.

- Close and seal the lid. Set on slow cook on low for two hours and stir every 30 minutes.
- When done, quick release the pressure. Spread onto a baking pan to cool and store in an airtight container.

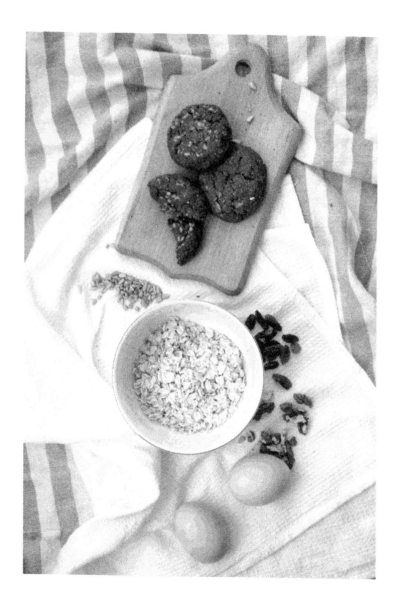

Chapter 10: Keto Diet Tips for Success

Cook large batches of food: While cooking can be greatly limited on the ketogenic diet with the addition of precooked meats and microwave-steamed vegetables, that doesn't mean you won't ever need to cook. Although, if you are limited on time or energy, cooking in large batches can save you energy, time, and money. Simply cook more food than you need and store it in the fridge or freezer. If you desire you can simply cook two or three servings at a time to store in the fridge, or you can make enough food to last you two or three weeks and store it in the freezer. This is wonderful for people on the go, as you simply have to remove it from the freezer and thaw it out in the microwave.

Budgeting for keto: Many people assume that following a keto diet will be expensive, but it really doesn't have to be. Your fat intake is going to be more than you are normally used to. Fats make you feel fuller for longer periods of time, unlike carbs. This means that you will be able to go longer between meals. When you aren't eating between meals, this works as another way to save money.

Since protein levels don't vary with the quality of the cut of meat, you aren't faced with buying expensive meats. Here are some other money-saving tips:

- Keep things simple. Your meals don't have to contain many different parts. The fewer ingredients you use, the less money you are going to be spending. If you make a simple omelet and have water with it, it is only going to cost you about $2.50. A Big Mac costs around $5.

- Buy fresh vegetables when they are in season. The rest of the year you can purchase frozen.

- You can usually get a better deal if you buy a whole chicken and cut it apart by yourself. Keep the carcass, too. This can be used to make bone broth which can help supplement loss of electrolytes.

- Watch for sales in your local grocery stores and stock up on these items, especially if you use a lot of them.

Eat more slowly: Early on when you are following the ketogenic diet, your body will still be figuring out how to best transform fat into fuel because it has rarely had to worry about such things before. As such, it can take you longer to feel full than would otherwise be the case because your body is still getting its new signals straight. While this is certainly nothing to worry about, when it is combined with the added hunger signals the body is sending out in hopes of being fed carbs, it can lead to scenarios where it is difficult to control yourself despite your best efforts.

While it is certainly natural to feel hungrier than normal during the early days of the keto diet it is important to resist the urge to tear through your meal as quickly as possible if you want to retain control. Eating more slowly will allow your body's signals to catch up to what is actually taking place which means you will start to feel full by the time you are finished and thus able to make smart choices with a clear head.

This can be something as simple as making an effort to chew each bite of food more than 10 times before swallowing. You should find this is enough to extend your meal past the point where your body can actually determine if you still need more fuel or are good for the time being. Other options include things like setting your utensils down between each bite of food or simply eating with others and enjoy the scenery and the company so that you have more options than just rushing through your meal to get back to whatever else it was you were doing.

Know your exact net carb limit: While you are going to want to stick to 15 or less net carbs per day when first entering ketosis, this is just to save you the hassle of determining the exact amount of net carbs that your body can handle. The fact of the matter is that each person is going to have a different net carb limit, which can also change over time. In order to provide yourself with all the data, you need to ensure that you have an accurate idea of just what is going on.

One of the most popular ways of doing so these days is through the use of the MyFitnessPal app which is one of the most popular calorie tracking apps around today, and with good reason. The base version is free, though some of the paid features are useful to those who are following the keto diet. The app also sets itself apart with the ease at which it is to share the progress. The app has a very large food database, but anyone can edit it, so it can sometimes be difficult to tell if the macros are reliable. Finally, the free version only tracks regular carbs, plus fiber, so you will have to do a little math as well.

If you are looking for something that is tailored to the keto diet specifically, then you may be interested in a Cronometer. While it costs $2.99, it comes with an officially curated food database which provides far more details about the foods you are considering putting into your body in addition to natively calculating keto macros.

Being able to precisely track what you are eating comes with numerous benefits on its own as well. First and foremost, you will find that you are able to exert willpower over what you are eating much more easily when you know you have to account for it specifically. Additionally, it will help you to get a more accurate picture of what you are consuming during the day as you will be surprised at how many small things you eat during the day that you don't think of as either eating a meal or snacking. Finally, it will help to ensure that you get in the habit of measuring the foods you eat until you have an accurate idea of what a true serving size is.

The role of fiber: Although fiber cannot be digested, it plays a key role in the digestion of carbohydrates in the body. It slows down the rate of digestion and absorption of carbohydrates, thereby preventing the blood sugar from rapidly shooting up. Aside from that, fibers provide food for your beneficial gut bacteria, improving digestion and bowel movement. It is also beneficial to ensure your fiber intake is right to aid in digestion and improve your bathroom habits. Fiber is essential for good bowel movements. Fiber also contains phytochemicals like lycopene, lutein, and indole-3-carbinol. These stimulate the immune system, fight free radicals, and protect and repair the DNA.

Be realistic: Keto diets are popular because of the quick slim down. This happens because your body releases a lot of water when it first begins using fat for energy. The scales are going to go down a few pounds and you might even look leaner. The first drop that you experience is usually only water weight. This doesn't mean that you haven't burned any fat. The main problem is, while studies have shown that you will lose weight, they haven't figured out if this is sustainable long term. Most people find that a strict eating plan is hard to stick to. If you do veer off the diet, you might gain all the weight back and then some.

Don't completely ignore calories: While following a ketogenic lifestyle means that you don't need to worry about counting calories as much as you would with many other diets, that doesn't mean you should ignore them completely. While an item that is high in healthy fat and contains a medium amount of protein and a small number of carbohydrates might look good on paper, if it also weighs in at 1,000 calories per serving then you are going to want to give it a wide berth no matter what. As such, it is helpful to have a general idea of the number of calories someone of your age, gender and lifestyle should try and consume in a given day and do your best to stay somewhere within the healthy zone. After all, just because you are going the extra mile to eat in a healthy fashion doesn't mean there is nothing else you can do to be more all-around healthy at all times.

Making it easier: The great thing about the keto diet is that it can be easily personalized for just about anybody. When you start, you can experiment with different things to see what will work best for you. There are some people that discover that they have to consume more fat in order to feel better, while there are others that can lower their carb intake more than others.

When you decide to start the ketogenic diet, try picking a time of the year where you don't have as much going on. Picking a slower time will give you the chance to focus solely on the diet and not everything else. Hectic times of the year, like the holidays, can cause more stress, but it can be done. One great way is to take your own keto friendly food. This is a good thing to do even after you have established yourself in the keto diet. Also, it would be a good idea to start on a Sunday or a Monday. Things just seem to work out better when you begin at the first of the week. You will likely find that it is a lot easier on the days where you have a lot going on because you won't have the time to think about food.

Another great way to keep from getting overwhelmed is to slowly introduce keto recipes. You'll notice that there will be a lot of ingredients that you probably haven't even heard of. Don't start out making those recipes. Start out with recipes that you know the ingredients of. With each passing week, add a new recipe to your routine.

Breakfast shouldn't be worried about too much. The majority of keto dieters don't even eat breakfast, or they have bulletproof coffee. If you do want to eat something, breakfast is the easiest meal to figure out. Simply scrambling some eggs in butter is a perfect keto meal. Lunch and dinners are very interchangeable so if you have leftovers from dinner, take those to work with your the next day for lunch. There's no sense in fretting over what to cook for lunch.

Include coconut or MCT oil: Not only does coconut oil provide you with many health benefits, but it contains many medium-chain triglycerides, also known as MCT oil. Consuming either coconut oil, or pure MCT oil can help increase ketone levels, energy, and satiety.

Unlike most other fats, medium-chain triglycerides have the ability to be rapidly digested and then delivered to the liver where they are used as fuel or transmuted into ketones. While you can buy pure MCT oil, coconut oil contains about fifty percent of medium-chain triglycerides, making it a wonderful health-promoting and energizing option. The remaining portion of coconut oil is lauric acid, which has also been shown in studies to produce a sustained level of ketones, therefore the coconut oil is a combination of two powerful fats for ketosis.

Coconut oil has also been shown in a wide range of studies to improve the symptoms of Alzheimer's disease, protect the nervous system, reduce the frequency of seizures in epileptics, and increase weight loss. Generally speaking, the more coconut oil you can successfully add to your diet in a day the better off you will be.

If you plan on adding coconut or MCT oil to your diet, it is a good plan to introduce them slowly so that your body can adjust. If you add these fats too quickly your digestive system will not be able to easily digest them, inducing possible diarrhea or stomach cramps. Thankfully, if you slowly start adding one teaspoon of coconut oil before eventually working up to two or three tablespoons over the course of a week or two, you shouldn't experience any digestive upset.

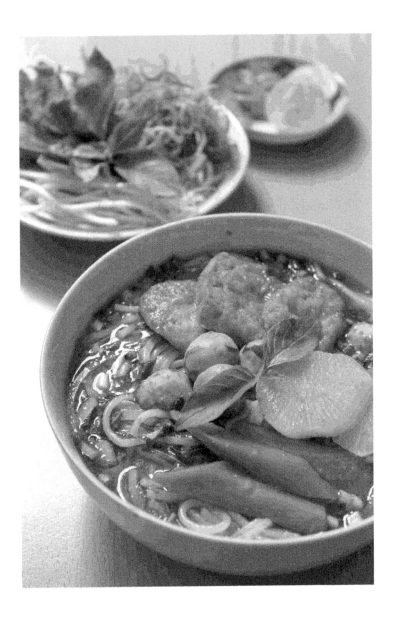

Conclusion

Thanks for making it through to the end of *Intermittent Fasting : The Ultimate Beginners Guide for Weight Loss, Burn Fat, Heal Your Body, Cure Illness With Intermittent Fasting and Ketogenic Diet*, let's hope it was informative and able to provide you with all of the tools you need to achieve your goals, whatever it is that they may be. Just because you've finished this book doesn't mean there is nothing left to learn on the topic, and expanding your horizons is the only way to find the mastery you seek.

Now that you have made it to the end of this book, you hopefully have an understanding of how to get started losing weight faster than ever before with a combination of the keto diet and intermittent fasting, as well as a strategy or two, or three, that you are anxious to try for the first time. Before you go ahead and start giving it your all, however, it is important that you have realistic expectations as to the level of success you should expect in the near future.

While it is perfectly true that some people experience serious success right out of the gate, it is an unfortunate fact of life that they are the exception rather than the rule. What this means is that you should expect to experience something of a learning curve, especially when you are first figuring out what works for you. This is perfectly normal, however, and if you persevere you will come out the other side better because of it. Instead of getting your hopes up to an unrealistic degree, you should think of your time spent fasting intermittently while following the keto diet as a marathon rather than a sprint which means that slow and steady will win the race every single time.

Finally, if you found this book useful in anyway, a review on Amazon is always appreciated!

Kathleen Moore

Made in the USA
Middletown, DE
10 June 2019